T0383700

The International Library of Psychology

PSYCHOANALYSIS AND BEHAVIOUR

Founded by C. K. Ogden

The International Library of Psychology

PSYCHOANALYSIS
In 28 Volumes

PSYCHOANALYSIS AND BEHAVIOUR

ANDRÉ TRIDON

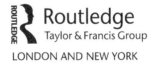

Routledge
Taylor & Francis Group
LONDON AND NEW YORK

First published in 1920
by Routledge
2 Park Square, Milton Park, Abingdon, Oxfordshire OX14 4RN
711 Third Avenue, New York, NY 10017

First issued in paperback 2014

Routledge is an imprint of the Taylor and Francis Group, an informa business

The publishers have made every effort to contact authors/copyright holders
of the works reprinted in the *International Library of Psychology*.
This has not been possible in every case, however, and we would
welcome correspondence from those individuals/companies
we have been unable to trace.

These reprints are taken from original copies of each book. In many cases
the condition of these originals is not perfect. The publisher has gone to
great lengths to ensure the quality of these reprints, but wishes to point
out that certain characteristics of the original copies will, of necessity, be
apparent in reprints thereof.

British Library Cataloguing in Publication Data
A CIP catalogue record for this book
is available from the British Library

Psychoanalysis and Behaviour
ISBN 0415-21108-5
Psychoanalysis: 28 Volumes
ISBN 0415-21132-8
The International Library of Psychology: 204 Volumes
ISBN 0415-19132-7

ISBN 13: 978-1-138-87571-5 (pbk)
ISBN 13: 978-0-415-21108-6 (hbk)

TABLE OF CONTENTS

Contents

PREFACE

This is an attempt at interpreting human conduct from the psychoanalytical point of view. The unconscious and involuntary play a tremendous part in human life, the more tremendous as they usually masquerade as conscious and voluntary. Courts and public opinion, disregarding that fact, either praise or condemn, either reward or punish. Psychoanalysis passes no judgments and only seeks to understand and help.

The author has not felt the necessity of restating historical and theoretical facts to which he devoted a previous book: "Psychoanalysis, its history, theory and practice." The various schools of analysis, however, having reached almost identical conclusions as to human behaviour, although they started from different premises, the last four chapters of the present book shall describe the paths followed by the four best known psychoanalysts, Freud, Jung, Adler and Kempf.

ANDRE TRIDON.

121 Madison Avenue,
New York City.   September 1920.

I. THE ORGANISM

CHAPTER I: THE UNCONSCIOUS

To the majority of people, our conscious life appears as the most important, if not the only important, form of life. Most of our rules of behaviour, most of our judgments on human actions are based upon that estimate of our conscious life.

And yet we are conscious of very few things at a time and we are conscious of each one of those things only for variable, some times, very short periods.

After a week, a day, an hour or a fraction of a second, the various things we were conscious of drop out of our consciousness, temporarily or permanently. We may witness a theatrical performance, be conscious of it that evening, think of it perhaps the next day, mention it several times in conversation, remember it years after when it is alluded to in our presence, and then "forget it."

But the impression made on us by that performance does not die off. It only becomes unconscious. That impression and millions of others are stored up in our "unconscious" where they continue to live as unconscious elements.

[13]

These impressions meant either active or passive reactions to certain stimulations, the yielding to or resistance to those stimulations, memory-images of satisfied cravings and of repressed cravings, joy or pain, longing or hatred, in other words, all our life from the day of our birth, with all its struggles against reality, its compromises with reality, its victories and defeats, etc.

All that past which we are constantly carrying with us and to which we are constantly adding, is bound, according to what elements predominate in it, to colour strongly our conscious view of life and to determine our conscious activities.

A neurologist, a sexual pervert, a sculptor and a manicure would react very differently to the sight of a woman's hand. An egotist would be unable to notice in his environment things of a neutral type, that is, unlikely to affect his egotism favourably or unfavourably. To a farmer, a certain accumulation of clouds might only suggest a danger to his crops; the same meteorological phenomenon might transport a painter with artistic joy. A chemist or a sailor would place a totally different construction on their observations of the same clouds.

We know that unconscious factors cause us to engage in certain forms of activity, to become insane, to fall asleep or to remain sleepless, to love a certain type and to remain frigid to another. They influence our methods of reasoning, making us at times illogical and one-sided, stubborn and unjust.

In other words our entire life is influenced, if not entirely determined, by unconscious factors.

Our unconscious is the greatest time and energy saving machine, provided it functions normally. Some of our simplest conscious acts presuppose an enormous amount of unconscious work. Stepping aside to dodge an automobile, simple as it appears, is only made possible by innumerable "mental" and "physical" operations such as realizing the nature, size, direction and speed, of the dangerous object, selecting a safe spot at a certain distance from it, performing the necessary muscular actions, etc., etc.

On the other hand we may, without any apparent reason, perform useless, absurd, harmful actions and be genuinely grieved or puzzled over our behaviour. We ask ourselves "What made me do that?"

Our unconscious made us do that. Our behaviour was dominated and determined by one or several factors unknown to us and which, unless investigated systematically, may remain unknown, puzzling, detrimental, if not dangerous, and may at some future time be once more the cause of irrational behaviour.

Our unconscious "contains" two sorts of "thoughts" : those which rise easily to the surface of our consciousness and those which remain at the bottom and can only be made to rise with more or less difficulty.

Our unconscious is like a pool into which dead leaves, dust, rain drops and a thousand other things are falling day after day, some of them floating on the surface for a while, some sinking to the bottom and, all of them, after a while, merging themselves with the water or the ooze. Let us suppose that two dead dogs, one of them weighted down with a stone, have been thrown into that pool. They will poison its waters, and people wishing to use those waters will have to rake the ooze and remove the rotting carrion. The dog whose body was not fastened to any heavy object will easily be brought to the surface and removed. The other will be more difficult to recover and if the stone is very heavy, may remain in the pool until ways and means are devised to dismember him or to cut the rope holding him down.

Another simile might be offered. Out of fifty persons assembled in a room, not one may be think-

[16]

ing of the multiplication table. Yet if some one points out three chairs worth six dollars a piece and asks the audience how much the three together are worth, the part of the multiplication table containing the answer shall rise to the surface of everybody's consciousness, to sink back into the unconscious a second later.

Other thoughts would not rise so willingly into consciousness: those associated with some painful or humiliating memory or with the repression of some human craving. Only a special effort aided by many association tests will in certain cases cut the rope that holds those "dead dogs tied to their paving stone."

Such thoughts are called complexes and they are the most disturbing element in our life, for, unknown to us, they exert a strong influence on all our mental operations and on our bodily activities.

It is not so much our consciousness as our unconscious which IS our personality. Our conscious thoughts are fleeting and changing, our unconscious is more permanent. If we take a list of some hundred words and ask a person to tell us what comes at once to his mind when he hears each word spoken, it will be noticed that the answers which come without any hesitancy would be the same several months afterward. Those answers, in fact,

[17]

by their wording, present a striking picture of the personality, a picture which only changes when the personality undergoes distinct modifications.

Only the words referring to the person's complexes are likely to change, as if the unconscious was trying to conceal the place where the "dead dogs" have been buried. In reaction tests, in fact, the subject's failure to give the same answer is taken to indicate a hidden complex. But even the varying answers given in such cases are closely related to one another.

When we remember how our unconscious has "grown," that is, through the accumulation of memories and repressions from the day of our birth, or even from our prenatal existence to the present day, we must realize that a large proportion of the elements which constitute it is primitive, infantile or childlike, unadapted or only partly adapted. Its influence on our behaviour is not likely, therefore, to facilitate our adaptation to the innumerable rules imposed by a more and more complex civilization.

Through all our life our unconscious follows us like the shadow of an archaic self, prompting us to seek a line of lesser resistance, or to give up the struggle with the modern world, to indulge ourselves in many ways which are no longer accept-

[18]

able socially; when childlike or infantile elements predominate in it, its influence may unfit us completely for life in modern communities unless we are brought to a clear realization of the ghostly power masquerading as ourselves and which tries to pull us back.

When the man we were yesterday offers us suggestions as to conduct, we are probably safe in accepting them. When the boy we were at 15, endeavours to convince us that his way was the only way, the struggle for mastery between ourselves and the boy may usher in a neurosis. When the infant we were at one or two years of age, coaxes us to indulge ourselves as he did and we yield to his entreaties, we may regress temporarily or permanently to a level at which we shall be adjudged insane.

Academic psychologists have suggested a number of very interesting but meaningless words to designate the varying degrees of unconsciousness, such as foreconscious, preconscious, subconscious, etc. . . .

For scientific purposes the word unconscious is sufficient. Instead of distinguishing degrees of unconsciousness which may easily change, it is preferable to assign reasons for unconsciousness. The multiplication table in the above illustration was unconscious because it was not needed, for reasons of economy. It became conscious when needed. Other factors, mentioned previously, remain unconscious because the thought of them is repressed or suppressed. Some are forgotten, because they are insignificant, some because the memory of them is weighted with unpleasant connotations as one of the dead dogs was weighted with a paving stone.

It is the task of psychoanalysis to make us thoroughly familiar with the content of our unconscious that we may on every occasion determine whether the voices talking to us from the past buried in us are the voices of civilization or the voices of regression.

Psychoanalysis forewarns us against any undue influence it may exert in the conduct of our lives and helps those of us who may have listened to the wrong voice to free themselves from their slavery.

Instead of saying, as academic psychologists would put it, that the psychoanalytic technique can make unconscious factors foreconscious and finally conscious we should say that it can establish a relation of cause-effect between certain acts and certain unconscious factors.

For that reason psychoanalysis is the only key to an understanding of human behaviour. Ethics

[20]

and statute books only record the various compromises which mankind in its onward march has had to make with reality. They have, however, no absolutely scientific value, because they are based upon the conception of an inexistent being, the average human being.

Psychoanalysis on the other hand discards the "average" man or woman and deals solely with the individual.

The neurotic applying for treatment who states that his case is a "very peculiar one" is both right and wrong. His case as a clinical picture is probably a very common one but as the content of one man's unconscious is necessarily very different from that of any other man's unconscious, no case can be prejudged from the observations made in any other case. Every case is "peculiar."

The law and current ethics criticize or punish a pool for containing a dead dog which is held down by a powerful weight, and for poisoning those who drink of its water.

Psychoanalysis looks for the corpse at the bottom of the pool and endeavours to remove it. Neither before nor after the operation does it pass judgments or pronounce sentences.

To understand is to forgive, but in spite of its frankly determinist attitude in matters of behaviour, psychoanalysis does not condone unethical or criminal behaviour. Hygienists would not insult or punish the infected pool but they would fence it off until the contaminating substances had been removed. Irrational and criminal individuals should be likewise restrained and isolated, not for purposes of castigation, but until such time when dangerous factors in their unconscious have been removed and when re-education has enabled them to resume their place among normal individuals.

BIBLIOGRAPHY

The subject of the unconscious is discussed very clearly in non-technical language by William Lay in "Man's Unconscious Conflict" (Dodd, Mead and Co.) pages 48 to 126.

This book is an excellent primer for those who wish to familiarize themselves with the terminology of psychoanalysis.

Advanced readers may study Jung's book "Psychology of the Unconscious" (Moffat Yard) which requires a certain knowledge of folklore, ancient religions and psychiatry.

The chapters on Instincts, Memory Images and Tropisms in Jacques Loeb's "Forced Movements, Tropisms and Animal Conduct" (Lippincott) will also prove very valuable from the mechanistic point of view.

CHAPTER II: BODY AND MIND, AN INDI-VISIBLE UNIT

Academic psychologists simplify their tasks by allotting the body to physiologists and occupying themselves exclusively with the mind. Applied psychology of the analytical type has been compelled to discard that arbitrary division of the human organism into "mental" and "physical." Physiologists prying their way into obscure "physical" phenomena have innumerable times reached a sort of middle kingdom in which it seems impossible to produce anything "physical" without producing at the same time something "mental," in which, to every "physical" stimulation, there corresponds a "mental" effect and to every "mental" stimulation corresponds a "physical" effect.

After observing the constant interrelation existing between secretions, attitudes and emotions, one no longer feels justified in speaking vaguely of the influence of the mind on the body or reciprocally. One can no longer understand life unless one admits that mind and body are one.

The task of the psychoanalyst would be a hope-

[23]

less one if he ever attempted to study the so-called "mental" disturbances as purely "psychic" phenomena; the physician who would treat bodily ailments as purely "physical" manifestations would be baffled and impotent.

It is only the profoundly ignorant who at the present day pretend to know the limits of the physical and of the mental and attempt to attribute certain phenomena to the mind and others to the body.

Cut off a frog's head, thereby removing the brain which is commonly supposed to be the seat of the mind, of the intelligence, of consciousness, etc. The frog then should be " entirely dead" or at least should not be expected to perform any act, except of a purely reflex type, showing any "intelligence." And yet if you apply a strong stimulus such as a drop of prussic acid to the skin of the frog's stomach, one of the legs will at once try to reach the burnt spot and to remove the harmful stimulus.

Such a "reflex" act proves that, even in the absence of any thinking apparatus, the organism is aware that something harmful is happening to one of its parts and endeavours to perform appropriate motions to protect itself against further destruction.

If a set of nerves and muscles can "think" as

[24]

clearly as that, unassisted by any brain or mind, the so-called purely physical must be endowed with a remarkable proportion of "mentality."

The deplorable inaccuracy of the words mental and physical is well illustrated by experiments made on dogs.

Feed a dog every possible morsel that will induce him to overeat until the beast turns in disgust from the most appetizing food.

Inject into that overfed dog blood from a dog who has been kept hungry for two days and the overfed dog will throw himself on food "as though" he were hungry.

The same experiment could probably be performed as successfully on a man. The man, however, would wonder at the possibility of his experiencing hunger after being surfeited with all sorts of dainties. He would doubt the testimony of his "senses," and speak of "nervous hunger," of "imaginary hunger," vague terms which explain nothing.

If a dog is infuriated by the presence of a cat, he will display for "reasons" which to him and the onlookers appear "plausible" and "logical," symptoms of anger such as the dilatation of his pupils, bristling of the hair, snarling, stiffening of the body, defensive poses.

Inject a small amount of adrenin into the veins of that dog or any other dog of not especially vicious disposition, and in the absence of any cat or any other disturbing element, he will, "without any reason" stare, snarl, bristle up his hair, and generally express, through threatening attitudes, violent anger.

When large amounts of adrenin are released into the human blood stream owing to the abnormal functioning of certain glands, set in motion perhaps by some obscure unconscious thought, a man may likewise assume an attitude of anger, "without any reason," and may justify his attitude by "imagining" a grudge against some people, or impatience at certain things. His attitude may later on appear to him absurd and incomprehensible. He may then excuse himself on the plea that "he lost control of himself" or "he was not himself."

A crowd may congregate and indulge in some ridiculous or violent deed of which, the following day, every individual member may feel deeply ashamed. "Crowd psychology," "mob suggestion" will then be invoked, the assumption being that all the individuals constituting the crowd had at one time a sort of "collective mind" dominated by one and the same obsessive "thought."

A curious light is thrown upon the behaviour of

[26]

mobs by the behaviour of copepods, small crusta-
ceans, when carbonated water or beer or alcohol
are poured into the aquarium in which they disport
themselves. As long as their water remains pure,
they are apparently in full possession of their
"free will" and displace themselves as they please.
As soon as the ingredients mentioned above are
added to the water, they all abandon their occupations and go to mass themselves at the end of the
aquarium which is turned toward the light.

If one continues to drop at intervals small quantities of carbonated or alcoholic liquids into the
aquarium, the little mob remains in the same position. It cannot turn round. Nor can the helpless
animals partake of their food, if that food happens
to be placed at the opposite end of the aquarium,
that is, away from the source of light.

Drain the polluted water or place the copepods
into fresh water and the mob will soon disperse,
each small animal regaining its freedom of individual motion and of direction.

Pour into the aquarium strychnin, caffein or
atropin and the copepods will once more gather
into a mob, this time, however, at the end of the
aquarium furthest removed from the light.

Their previous "fondness" for sunlight has been
replaced by a "craving" for darkness.

[27]

Prophets, artists, reformers, lovers, may undergo all sorts of trials, brave starvation and death in order to seek their ideal, and some day they may forsake their ideal. Lovers having recovered from their "infatuation" may recall with astonishment or shame many absurd things they said or did once and look upon their former love object with disgust or even hatred.

Certain animals like copepods can be fooled a number of times and be made to fall in love now with the sun, now with the darkness. Others which, were they human beings, would be said to learn very quickly from experience, are never victimized but once by their "idealistic cravings" and afterward lead a perfectly "sensible" life.

Take some newly hatched caterpillars and deposit them at the foot of a rod or stick on which the sunlight is shining. They will all climb to the top and stay there, staring at the sun, apparently engrossed in the contemplation of their "ideal." In fact they would starve to death unless some one fed them a small piece of green leaf.

As soon as they partake of that food, their obsessive sun worship seems to disappear. They climb down the barren stick and seek other stores of food, never bothering any more with the sun or other sources of light.

[28]

Watch the behaviour of bees at mating time. Male and female can only fly in one direction, that is toward the sun, and their amorous ecstasy carries them into "higher regions," "uplifts" them, takes them "far from the earth." The sexual act performed, they both become once more creatures of the earth, fly back to their native hive and no longer feel the "fascination of the empyrean."

An invention described recently in publications devoted to electrical science shows how difficult it would be to draw an absolute line of demarkation between actions apparently due to physical and chemical causes and actions apparently due to the exercise of our "will power" and prompted by "feelings," etc.

The electric dog has two eyes supplied with condensing lenses focussed on two selenium cells. Selenium is an element whose electrical properties change under the influence of light. The selenium cells control two electro-magnetic switches. Two motors, on the right and left, can propel the dog forward or backward.

When light, as for instance from a small flash lamp, is thrown on both eyes, the current is switched on to both motors and the dog advances toward the light. When the lamp is held to the right, the right motor only is actuated and the dog turns to the right. The dog follows the light in the most complicated manœuvres. Shade the light and the dog stops; reverse the motors and the dog runs away from the light, dodging it wherever it may come from.

Thus a moth will rush toward a flame, thus owls fly in distress from any bright light, thus human beings are perhaps "propelled" toward a goal, which they think they are striving for, thus the races of the earth once started on their westward wanderings, thus cities and towns, when not restrained by natural obstacles of an insuperable nature, like mountains or bodies of water, spread to the westward.

Naturalists manage to make the problem a little more complicated by telling us that animals and plants which are "fond" of light, that is which are involuntarily and unavoidably determined by light, are also "fond" of blue and green, while animals which are negatively heliotropic, that is "fond" of darkness and afraid of light, are "fond" of the colour red.

And experiments on thousands of human beings have revealed that men are most deeply affected by blue, women by red.

Whenever experiments first made on animals

[30]

have been tried on human beings their results have been found to confirm the first observations.

We know that the same method of training makes both a man and a passenger pidgeon sexual perverts. Laboratory experiments have proved that female cats and female dogs react more slowly to anger stimuli than the males of both species, the result being a smaller percentage of sugar found in their urine. Observations made on college students of both sexes prove that the rule holds good when human beings are concerned. Human subjects, unfortunately, cannot be used as frequently as they should be to assure us of the universal application of certain biological and biochemical laws.

Some day when we abandon our wasteful method of dealing with criminals and give unredeemable offenders an opportunity to pay for the damage they have inflicted by submitting to scientific experiments likely at times to result in death, we may be able to ascertain accurately in what measure chemical determinism, for example, rules the lives of men.

Specialization being the only road to thorough knowledge and efficiency, body and mind must at present, for the sake of convenience, be treated separately when in distress. Internist and analyst, however, must co-operate, both applying the latest

[31]

methods devised in their particular field and submitting to each other the doubtful details of every case.

While analysts agree that innumerable diseases of the so-called physical variety are induced or invited by some unconscious predisposing factor, no analyst denies the value of medical help or would suggest doing without it. If a subject has been so weakened by a wrong mental attitude that his body has become an easy prey for certain bacilli, all efforts should be made to check or eliminate those bacilli in order to avoid the further inroads they might make on the organism.

Specific medical treatment should be sought under the direction of a physician who keeps himself well informed as to the latest therapeutic methods, the most efficient pharmaceutic preparations, etc. The family physician, the surgeon, the average specialist, however, cannot be expected to follow all the research work done in applied psychology.

Although Freud and other prominent analysts have stated that psychoanalytical practitioners need not have medical training, an analyst should possess a good working knowledge of anatomy, physiology and neurology. Reciprocally, every physician should receive some elementary training in applied

[32]

psychology, regardless of whether he is to take up the practice of general medicine or to specialize in some particular branch of the medical profession.

Then, those who treat the more obviously material part of the organism and those who treat the more intangible part of the personality can co-operate intelligently in relieving the ailments of the human unit.

BIBLIOGRAPHY

Two books are absolutely essential to readers desiring to study the problem of the interrelations of body and mind from the modern physiological point of view. Loeb's book mentioned in the bibliography for the preceding chapter and W. B. Cannon's capital work "Bodily Changes in Pain, Hunger, Fear and Rage" (Appleton). The latter book contains a very readable and entertaining summary of many experiments made by Cannon and his students not only on laboratory animals but on themselves as well, showing the chemical changes which correspond to the various "emotions." G. W. Crile's "Man an Adaptive Mechanism," while not as recent as Cannon's book, should also be consulted.

CHAPTER III: NERVES AND NERVOUS-NESS

Nerves, nervous and nervousness are terms which should be used less frequently and less carelessly. "My nerves are on edge" or "I am a nervous wreck" are picturesque expressions devoid of any meaning and which convey a very inaccurate picture of what is taking place in the organism.

To the layman, nerves are just nerves; the nerve which a dentist "kills" and the nerve which makes our heart palpitate are to him identical things.

In reality there are in the human body two nervous systems whose appearance, colour, make up, distribution and functions are as different as night is from day.

There is the sensori-motor system, or the system of nerves which bring to the brain the information about the condition of the various parts of the body and about the way in which those parts are affected by the environment: the nerves which tell us what the eye "sees," what the mouth "tastes," what the nose "smells," whether the water in which we poke

[34]

our toe is cold or hot, whether the apple we hold is hard or soft.

That system also transmits from the brain to the various muscles definite orders based upon the information received. Motor nerves open or close our eyes, cause us to chew or spit out certain kinds of food, to extend our arm toward a desirable object or withdraw it from a dangerous object, etc.

The sensori-motor nerves are white fibres enveloped in a fatty sheath interrupted at intervals by nodes.

Besides this system there is another nervous system for which various names are being used, such as the vegetative system, the sympathetic system or the autonomic system. These nerves are white fibres covered by a very thin membrane instead of a thick sheath and presenting a more regular appearance owing to the absence of nodes.

Instead of issuing directly from the spinal column as the sensori-motor nerves do, the autonomic nerves, with the exception of the vagus which has its root in the brain, take their roots in a column of ganglia located in front of the vertebrae.

Although this system disintegrates soon after death, for it is poorly protected and its ganglia lie close to tissues which putrefy readily (nasal mu-

[35]

cous membrane, buccal cavity and intestinal canal), it is older than the sensori-motor system and it is fully developed at birth.

The autonomic system supplies the internal organs of the body, tear glands, sweat glands, salivary glands, hair roots, lungs, heart, stomach, liver, intestine, adrenal glands, bladder, rectum and genitals. It carries motor impulses, but scientists are not agreed as to whether it carries sensations. It also controls in part the movements of the pupil.

The autonomic system is divided up into two subsystems which we shall designate as the craniosacral division or end division and the thoracicolumbar division, or sympathetic division or middle division.

The two divisions are absolutely antagonistic in action. For instance the cranio-sacral contracts the pupil, the sympathetic dilates it; the cranio-sacral division slows down the heart action, the sympathetic division accelerates it.

The cranio-sacral division promotes all the activities which build up the individual and assure the continuance of the race.

The sympathetic division which extends from the neck to the upper sacral region, decreases or stops all those activities in emergencies and releases safety devices.

[36]

For instance the cranio-sacral division causes saliva to flow, which helps the disintegration of food in the mouth; it causes the stomach glands to secrete gastric juice and the stomach to contract regularly and vigorously, which activates the digestion and speeds the digested food on its way into the intestine; it contracts the intestine and hence assists the elimination of waste matter; it holds the rectum and bladder openings closed until the proper accumulation of feces or urine makes voiding necessary; it regulates the heart beats, prevents the pupil from admitting too much light and focuses it so that it throws a clear image on the retina; finally it fills the exterior genitals with blood and enables them to perform their specific functions.

The sympathetic division, on the contrary, stops the flow of saliva and of gastric juice, stops the contractions of the stomach or reverses their direction, so that food may be regurgitated into the aesophagus and, at times, vomited; it speeds the heart action; at times, it voids suddenly the bladder and bowels; releases into the blood stream a flow of adrenin which contracts the arteries and a flow of sugar from the liver which supplies the body with extra fuel; stops all genital functions; causes the pupil to dilate, thus giving the eye a staring glare; bristles the hair, causing goose flesh, etc.

[37]

One can see at once how all the activities of the sympathetic protect the organism either directly, by initiating necessary activities, or indirectly, by inhibiting certain activities which are not necessary in emergencies.

When the organism is in danger, that is, must resort to fight or flight, nutrition and sex activities should cease. Not only should they cease because the organism in danger cannot attend to them properly, but also because they deflect toward their specific organs a certain amount of blood which is needed elsewhere for defensive purposes. Hence the dry mouth, the arrested gastric action, the impotence induced by fear.

As the blood must circulate freely in the endangered organism and absorb as much oxygen as possible, the heart beats are increased and so is the rate of respiration. As a larger amount of energy has to be expended, the glycogen (sugar) stored up in the liver must be released into the blood stream, after the fashion of a motorist who "steps on the gas" in order to climb a steep hill; if a wound be sustained, adrenin is mixed with the blood causing it to coagulate more quickly and close the wound; finally the hair must be raised, affording to certain animals, such as cats and dogs, a certain amount of protection against teeth and claws and surround-

[38]

ing the body, in the case of porcupines and hedge-hogs, with an impassable barrier of sharp daggers.

The sudden voiding of the bowels and bladder caused by fright is another emergency measure taken by the sympathetic division. Empty bowels and an empty bladder present a more favourable condition in the case of deep abdominal injuries, while the same organs, if full, might cause complications.

The activities of the sympathetic division correspond to what we may call the *safety urge,* while the cranial division which promotes nutrition and assimilation would correspond to the *food-ego-power urge* and the sacral division to the *sex urge.*

We may notice that the nerves of ego and sex work in unison.

The two divisions of the autonomic system are not always balanced with perfect accuracy and one of them is bound to predominate. This will enable us to distinguish roughly three "nervous" types.

The type in which the positive activities which build up the individual and further the continuance of the race are not hampered by the negative activities of the sympathetic except in emergencies.

This is the type we may justly consider as normal.

The second type is one in which the positive

activities are so strong that they cannot be checked in emergencies by the safety nerves. When the personality is overwhelmed by the cranio-sacral division, that is by the ego and sex urges, the individual is unadaptive and unsocial. Criminal, gluttonous, obscene imbeciles belong to that type for which the terms vagotonic has been suggested.

In the third type, or sympathicotonic type, the sympathetic division functions in and out of season, flashing danger signals when there is no danger and holding back the natural cravings for nutrition, self-expression, acquisition, power, reproduction, etc. Neurotics suffering from anxiety, obsessions, phobias, nervous indigestion, psychic impotence, etc., belong to this type.

A very simple test has been devised to determine to what type a subject belongs. It is known as the Aschner test. It is based on the fact that the ends of both divisions, the cranial and the sympathetic divisions, can be reached and stimulated by pressure on the pupil.

The cranial division increases the heart beats and the sympathetic division decreases them. By applying the same stimulation to both divisions, the one which is more powerful will react more easily than the other. If after pressing on the eyeballs for half a minute, the initial pulse, let us say 90,

[40]

has been reduced to about 80, the patient is probably normal. If the pulse rate has been decreased by more than 10 or 12 beats, the patient is vagotonic, and if the pulse rate has remained unchanged or has been increased the patient is sympathicotonic.

A study of the autonomic system enables us to visualize complexes as defensive actions of the sympathetic division or safety urge which were initiated at some past time, generally in infancy when stimuli are likely to produce the deepest impression and which continue to be performed when no actual danger has to be warded off, or in emergencies which are not real emergencies but appear as such owing to wrong associations.

A child, frightened unwisely, may all his life show defence and fear reactions, which means that the nerves of his sympathetic division will constantly interfere with his digestion, his heart action, his intestinal peristalsis, his sex life.

A child hurt by a doctor with a black beard, a classical case in psychoanalytic literature, unconsciously associated in later life all men with black beards with the man who hurt him once and when meeting such a man suffered from arterial tension connected with fright.

Experiments made on dogs illustrate well the mechanism of association.

[41]

A dog was submitted to a delicate operation whereby the gastric juice secreted by his stomach would run into a graduated tube. For several days a bell was rung every time the dog was given food. To the sight of food there always corresponded a flow of gastric juice. One day the bell was rung but no food was offered to the animal. In spite of the absence of food, gastric juice began to trickle into the test tube. A "bell association" had been created in the dog's organism. In other words, as for several days the sound of a bell had been connected with the sight and taste of food, his autonomic nerves promoted the flow of gastric juice as soon as the bell rang.

A study of the autonomic activities sheds a new light upon many actions which at the present day are considered as voluntary and subjected to criticism or praised from a purely ethical point of view based upon the distinction between body and mind.

A sixty candle power bulb should not be criticized for carrying an amount of electrical power inferior to that which can flow through a hundred candle bulb.

A coward is not a coward because he wishes to run away, but because his sympathetic nerves promoting flight are especially sensitive to fright stimuli which in other men would produce no reaction or a reaction of fight. As Jacques Loeb would put it, a coward runs in the direction where his legs carry him. As the unscientific layman would express it, the coward "loses his nerve" or "is all nerves" or "cannot control his nerves."

Punishing a coward and insulting him will not make him a brave man. It may compel him to pretend for a time that he is brave, after which he may succumb to shell-shock when his cravings for safety, long repressed, assert themselves violently and abnormally.

But he need not remain a coward and can be trained to master his fear by analyzing it and by disintegrating the absurd associations which set his organism in flight when no dangerous emergency exists.

A coward with a well developed intelligence can be made, through education, as indifferent to certain fear stimuli as other people can be made indifferent to some apparently alarming symptoms of sickness.

For example: any one taking the typhoid vaccine will after the first injection feel dreadfully sick. He will develop violent fever, suffer from headaches, thirst, palpitations, nausea, he will feel very weak, etc., in other words, he will, within twenty-four hours, experience most of the symptoms of the

[43]

disease against which the vaccine is to protect him. Duly warned by a physician, the patient will not worry over those disturbances which are "expected," as suppuration is expected after vaccination for smallpox.

The patient knows what is causing his malaise and what its duration shall be. While he could not very well "enjoy" the situation, he resigns himself to it as to something temporary and unavoidable.

On the other hand, should a careless physician fail to warn the patient of the effects of the first hypodermic dose, the patient would add to the unpleasant condition induced by the vaccine a deep worry, a fear of possible complications and perhaps devise unnecessary plans for emergency action, thereby affecting his heart beats, his gastric and intestinal activities and so on.

Knowing to what type he belongs is as necessary for a human being as knowing, for instance, whether one of his legs is shorter than the other. A cripple in ignorance of the disparity of his legs, would gather the impression that the road he was travelling was strewn with ruts and obstructions. The longer leg would seemingly encounter numberless obstacles while the shorter would be constantly descending into holes.

[44]

The man with a vagotonic tendency whose ego and sex urges are apt to disregard the warnings of his safety urge and the man with a sympathicotonic tendency whose sympthetic division is constantly raising the danger flag are bound to have very distorted impressions of their mental states and of their environment.

Knowing themselves better, they can discount considerably such deceptive impressions and thereby correct their behaviour.

Those called upon to judge them can also by understanding better their nervous mechanism, help them to conform to standard conduct.

Even the perfectly normal man can derive much comfort from knowing positively that he is normal at times when, in a crisis or emergency, he might conceive doubts as to his condition. A knowledge of the functioning of one's autonomic system is at all times of great assistance in remaining normal.

That knowledge also enables one to adopt or to avoid for scientific, that is, plausible and compelling reasons, certain forms of behaviour.

The following observation made on dogs by Pavlof teaches a lesson which should be remembered by every human being.

A dog submitted to the surgical operation I mentioned previously secreted some seventy cubic centimetres of gastric juice when fed a certain amount of meat. One day, a cat was brought into the laboratory while he was partaking of his meal and aroused his anger. On that occasion, the amount of gastric juice which flowed into the test tube was just one tenth that accompanying a peaceful undisturbed meal. Anger and fear had raised the danger signal in his organism and prepared the dog for fight or flight, but not for the enjoyment of a meal.

A quarrel at the dinner table affects human beings as the sight of a cat affected our dog. Their flow of gastric juice is stopped or considerably reduced and whatever food they take into their stomachs would linger in that organ much longer than it should normally. The result will be some form of "nervous indigestion," perhaps nausea and in extreme cases, vomiting.

Observations of a similar order were made on a small boy suffering from a gastric fistula which allowed gastric juice to flow out of his body. When the boy chewed pleasant food, the flow was copious, whereas the chewing of some unpleasant or indifferent substance was not followed by any secretion.

The flow of gastric juice is not induced solely, as many people think, by the pleasant taste of food.

[46]

The mere sight of appetizing aliments is sufficient to start the digestive fluids.

Hence, a meal served in an attractive dining room, on clean linen, in dainty dishes, with flowers on the table, in a peaceful, soothing atmosphere, to the tune of caressing, unemotional music, is likely to be digested more easily than food served in slovenly, noisy surroundings.

This applies to almost every experience in life.

Pleasant memories of gratifying happenings create durable associations, like the food-bell association which had such an appetizing effect on Pavlof's dog. Unpleasant memories produce perhaps even more lasting effects of the opposite character and are responsible for a thousand "nervous" ills.

Every psychological theory will have to be revised according to the rather recent findings of scientists touching the autonomic functions. While space does not allow us to dwell at length on that aspect of the subject, we may say a few words on the new interpretation of will-power which can be based upon the study of the autonomic nervous system.

The vagotonic, whose "animal" activities can hardly be checked by a weaker sympathetic division, is called "a creature of instinct," "led by his cravings," "subservient to his lower nature," "lacking in will-power," etc.

He whose sympathetic system acts in all emergencies and in emergencies only, that is, does not create absurd, unconscious reasons for illogical behaviour, is credited with a great amount of will-power.

He whose sympathetic system acts in and out of season, overpowering his ego and sex urges, creating emergencies and raising obstacles, is constantly "nervous," vacillating, considering one course and then another, "unable to make up his mind."

Education undertaken by a trained psychologist, not by a disciplinarian, may alter the first type by developing in his sympathetic division a fear of the absolute privation which may be the consequence of vagotonic indulgence.

The third type also can be trained to recognize a true emergency from an imaginary one and to gauge accurately the size of the obstacles rising in his path.

Neither type should be dealt with by jailers or judges. Neither should be held responsible for behaviour due to weakness or self-deception. Both should, if their conduct is socially intolerable, be restrained and educated. Those whose nervous

[48]

system appears inadaptable should remain the wards of the state and be considered as victims of organic maladjustment for which they are in no wise responsible.

BIBLIOGRAPHY

The subject of nerves cannot be well understood unless the reader makes himself familiar with the autonomic nervous system which in the majority of medical books is designated as the sympathetic system.

The most important publication on the subject is H. Higier's "Vegetative Neurology" (Nervous and Mental Disease Pub. Co.) which is very technical. Consult also M. Laignel Lavastine's "The Internal Secretions and the Nervous System" (Nervous and Mental Disease Pub. Co.) and Cannon's previously mentioned work.

G. V. N. Dearborn's "The Influence of Joy" (Little Brown) and L. E. Emerson's "Nervousness" (Little Brown), are two small books casting interesting sidelights on the subject.

II. PROBLEMS OF CHILDHOOD

CHAPTER I.   CHILDHOOD FIXATIONS

The seed of all mental disturbances is sown in our childhood years.   Whether we hold with Freud that childhood memories, habits and repressions disturb our mental balance in later years, or assume with Adler that the neurotic adult simply draws upon his childhood memories for the woof of his fancies, the fact remains that one's childhood, directly or indirectly, determines the content and form of one's neurosis.

The problems of childhood are therefore the problems of the adult.   To a normal, happy childhood corresponds a normal, happy adulthood. We cannot state that to an abnormal, unhappy childhood there always corresponds an abnormal unhappy adulthood, for most people manage to remain normal regardless of what they do or have to suffer at the hands of others; but we can state that to every abnormality observed in an adult corresponds some abnormal situation which dominated the subject's childhood.

The most fateful complication in a child's life and one whose consequences are recognized by

[53]

analysts of all schools without any exception, is what Freud has designated as the Oedipus complex, or the excessive attachment of a child for the parent of the opposite sex, resulting in a more or less violent dislike of the parent of the same sex.

Freud called it the Oedipus Complex as an illusion to the well known legend of Oedipus, King of Thebes, who killed his father Laius and married his mother Jocasta.

Students of ancient religions and folk lore have noticed that the conflict between father and son, mother and daughter, constitutes the substance of thousands of mythological or popular legends. Psychiatrists have observed it re-appearing in many forms of mental derangement.

Freud has stated that such an excessive attachment or "fixation" is unconsciously incestuous.

The Swiss school of analysts would rather believe that the fixation is purely symbolical, the boy selecting his mother, the girl, her father, as an ideal of authority, intelligence, power, etc.

Adler, of Vienna, on the other hand, believes that the incest situation is imagined by the neurotic as one of the components of his regression to a period of his life when he was absolutely dependent on one of the parents and did not have to face life and its struggles.

[54]

None of those three views should exclude the others. There may be a slightly sensuous attachment in certain cases, encouraged by caresses of the mother for the son and of the father for the daughter, in which there is a slight amount of veiled sexuality, each of the parents showing preference for the child of the opposite sex. But in many cases, Jung's and Adler's views appear very plausible.

To those three hypotheses we may add a fourth one: Imitation is probably the most potent factor in human and animal life. Like instinct, it probably resolves itself into a set of little understood physical, chemical and nervous phenomena, some of which have been elucidated only recently.

We are what we are because we have imitated some man or woman whose mannerisms, attitudes, mode of speech, and consequently, whose emotional life we have unconsciously reproduced.

As in the first years of our life we have no one to imitate but our parents, our parents are likely to become our most obsessing model or ideal.

This phenomenon presents many dangers. The normal child would be one who, up to the time of puberty, had imitated both parents without showing much partiality (admitting of course that the parents harmonized well enough not to create a conflict in the child's mind); who at puberty, would imitate the parent of the same sex, without exhibiting any hostility toward the parent of the opposite sex; and who finally would select secondary imitation objects outside of the family circle, thus building up a consistent and original personality.

The parental traits would be there, father and mother contributing varied qualities, and outsiders furnishing pleasing variations upon the parental type, introducing into the blend no discordant features.

There are too many cases, however, in which that happy situation is disturbed. Sickness in childhood may bring one child under the constant influence of one parent to the almost complete exclusion of the other; and so may the death or continued absence of one of the parents. One of the parents may for rather regrettable reasons, attract and amuse the child; a neurotic, eccentric parent will have more influence upon his children than his normal mate (circus freaks attract children more than athletes), etc.

Children coming home from the circus almost invariably imitate the freaks or the clowns, but even Freud would fail to drag a sexual explanation into that "fixation" which is often of long duration and incredibly powerful, considering the short time

[56]

in which the children were exposed to the influence of their favourites.

Three hours at the circus may mean several weeks of attempts at performing certain stunts. A little boy of my acquaintance walked for several weeks like Charlie Chaplin after seeing him once.

In many cases, the Oedipus situation resolves itself then into an exaggerated imitation of one parent by the child.

A boy having selected his mother as the most perfect model, is bound to dislike his father who, not only is so unlike her, but wields too much influence over her.

If, on the contrary, he had selected his father as his exclusive model, he would dislike his mother, who is unlike the father and dominates him in certain respects.

The family romance of the neurotic girl would be similar to that of the neurotic boy.

Imitation explains as much as sexuality and rids certain details of the romance of their apparently sexual aspect.

The boy with a fixation on his mother, who constantly fondles her and has to be taken into her bed, is not attracted by any of his mother's physical qualities. He is, in all respects but one, a female who feels no embarrassment in close contact with another female and does not expect her to feel any embarrassment either. The sexual fate of such boys, who later in life are very indifferent to women and not infrequently passive homosexuals, confirms the suspicion that it is rather imitation of the mother and self-identification with her than repressed incest cravings which dominate their behaviour.

The many male and female neurotics who are attracted solely to married men and women are subjects with strong fixations who seek, not primarily one physical or mental type for which they have a special affinity, but a situation, which in their childhood years was normal and habitual. The father they loved had a wife, the mother they loved had a husband.

Their jealousy of their lover's wife or of their mistress's husband is what their dislike of the unloved parent was, not sexual but egotistical.

The boy with a mother fixation and the girl with a father fixation, will not only try to be like the favourite parent, but will on all occasions try to be as unlike the unloved parent as possible. (Clergymen's sons.)

One boy I have observed was the son of a professional man, very conservative, prudish and snobbish to a degree.

[58]

His mother fixation had been nursed along by too much petting and fondling. At sixteen he still played in mother's bed mornings and evenings. At eighteen he showed absolutely no interest in girls and compared every girl he knew to his mother in a way most disadvantageous to the girl.

After a severe crisis at the time of puberty when he once attempted suicide, his opposition to every one of his father's ideas and plans for his future began to manifest itself very clearly.

The father was extremely conservative; the son embraced readily all radical beliefs. The father was conventional, the son unconventional in his behaviour and speech, and very slovenly in his way of dressing. The father was very settled in his habits, the son led the most irregular life, sleeping all day and loafing all night, having his meals at all times of the day or night.

His revolt against the father-image, symbolical of authority, caused him to be involved in difficulties with various teachers and finally to leave college.

In his sedulous avoidance of the father type he shunned all professional people and spent most of his time with menials and labourers.

His distaste for work, which prevented him from holding a position for more than a few days at a time, was in part an imitation of the comparative idleness of his middle class mother, financially dependent on his father, and in part an expression of dislike of his employers symbolizing the father's authority, and also a way of "getting even" with his father.

His constant schemes for getting-rick-quick and his passion for gambling were attempted flights from reality and a search for the line of least effort.

The struggle between his normal and his abnormal tendencies revealed itself in his variable attitude to his mother whom he at times overwhelmed with caresses and at times treated very scornfully.

Another neurotic with a decided fixation on his mother was unable to enjoy any food which had not been prepared by her or according to her recipes. Dishes which had never been served in his home during his childhood repelled him and when courtesy compelled him to eat of them, he generally developed nausea and vomiting. In this case, the mother fixation had not had any crippling effects as far as sexual cravings were concerned. He consorted with many women of different types but selected for his wife a woman of the mother type whom he constantly taunted by instituting unpleasant comparisons between her and his mother.

[60]

This man always voiced a frank hatred of his father and like the preceding type indulged constantly in dreams of get-rich-quick schemes which his restlessness never allowed to mature.

Besides heterosexual fixations or fixations on the parent of the opposite sex, we must consider homosexual fixations or fixations on the parent of the same sex.

They do not lead to conflicts as acute as those precipitated by the Oedipus situation. The boy with a father fixation is not impelled by his dislike of his mother to seek forms of behaviour which are eccentric or absurd, for, being a male, he will on all occasions act in ways different from hers. His dislike will be due to her dissimilarity to his ideal, which he will consider as an inferiority.

Very different from the boy with a mother fixation, the boy with a father fixation will not shun women but he will despise them and fear them. They will attract him as they attract the father he imitates but he will be more or less ashamed of yielding to their attraction. He will love them and torture them and the origin of many cases of cruel sadism is generally to be traced back to such a situation.

Both forms of fixation have a crippling influence on a human being's life. Clinging too closely to

[61]

an ideal, he has a tendency to disparage all conditions which differ from the conditions under which he acquired a fixation.

The man with a mother fixation will regret the days when he still was his mother's little boy; when life's emergencies threaten him with defeat he may regress to the childhood level on which he then lived.

The man with a father fixation will follow the same deceptive line of least effort; there will be a difference, however. While the man with a mother fixation is likely to be a rebel, the man with a father fixation is generally a crusty conservative, a neophobiac, ranting over the good old days, old fashioned in every way, at times more conservative even than his father, for his father may have grown mentally while he lingers in the stage during which he acquired his fixation and still imitates his father as his father was when he himself was from five to fifteen years old.

A conflict between the parents results often in a severe conflict in the child's organism. Parents living in disharmony lack fairness, measure and dignity. Their hostility to each other makes them repellent to the child who is constantly in doubt as to whom to imitate. In certain cases a fixation

[62]

on one of the parents may have disastrous effects. B. M.'s parents never agreed and finally separated. B. M. realized her mother's mental inferiority and drew farther and farther away from her in childhood. She was extremely attracted by her neurotic father whose lack of kindness and erratic ways, on the other hand, repelled her. Her psychology has ever since been complicated by the following speculation: "I shall do this because my father would have done it but it is wrong for me to do it for my father was an unworthy type." The result has been acute hysterical suffering.

I shall mention in the chapter on the Love Life the various perversions due to maladjustments of the fixation type in childhood.

From a consideration of the mental growth of the child, one is forced to accept the conclusion that the presence of a male and a female in the household is absolutely necessary if the offspring is to be normal in later life. The child brought up by only one parent is likely to be one-sided or perverse.

Affectionate parents are a source of great danger for their children and so are those who do not know how to restrain their children's affection when it gets out of bounds.

[63]

Indifferent parents or the removal of the parents by death in the child's infancy cripple the child in another way.

Egotism of the positive, progressive, creative type is the most valuable human trait, the trait which differentiates man from the animals. A certain amount of self-love, self-confidence, self-reliance is absolutely necessary in life.

The child whom no parent has praised and who has been treated like an intruder, the orphan committed to some institution where teachers or keepers, however kind they may be, cannot lavish on fifty or a hundred children the love which individual parents would lavish on each of them separately, suffer from a certain sense of inferiority which often leads to negativism.

Such children do not know that they are important for they have never seemed important to any one. When herded in institutions they only have distant models for imitation, the few adults they could imitate being strangers separated from them by a wall of indifference. The result is often a stunting in mental and physical growth due to the wholesale imitation of children by children.

The solution of the fixation problem will not be within our reach until the phenomenon of imitation has been studied more completely. At present a

few scattered observations made by biologists constitute the only material at our disposal. Those
few and unrelated facts, however, are enough to
make us suspect the tremendous importance of
imitation as a factor in human development.

CHAPTER II. THE SEXUAL ENLIGHTEN-MENT OF CHILDREN

One of the statements made by Freud and which exposed him to the bitterest criticism on the part of hostile or ill-informed opponents, was that in children, even for the tenderest age, the sexual life attains a much greater degree of development than was generally conceded and that its growth is gradual and continuous from the day of birth. Puberty is the culmination of that progressive ripening instead of being, as it is considered by many, the sudden, unprepared outburst of the sexual instinct.

Sexual, urinary and fecal activities being controlled by the same nerves develop along parallel lines. All of them, however, are submitted to a severe regulation which in the case of sex amounts to almost complete repression.

In probably many more cases than parents and nurses are willing to admit, there is a certain amount of sexual self-gratification indulged in by children between the ages of three and five, that is, long before puberty. Much of it certainly escapes observation.

[66]

Whatever of it is observed is usually considered by the average parent as a manifestation of some "vicious" tendency, and is repressed either by threats and punishment or by mechanical means such as binding the children's hands at night, etc.

The general opinion at the present day in scientific circles is that infantile onanism is simply one of nature's primitive ways of developing the child's sexual powers, a process to be watched closely by the parents and stopped if indulged in excessively by immobilizing the child's hands, but under no circumstances to be repressed by threats or punishment.

To that period of infantile onanism corresponds naturally one of intense and stubborn curiosity on the part of the child about matters pertaining to reproduction. That curiosity is generally brought to its climax by the arrival of a baby either in the family or in a house of the neighbourhood and the child will have no peace until he knows "where babies come from."

What shall parents do when such a question is put to them? The problem is simpler and yet more complicated than it seems at first.

The question is not: "Must children be told?" but "Who shall tell them and how?"

If every grown up will be honest with himself

he will have to confess that as soon as he attended a kindergarten or school his sexual enlightenment(?) was begun by the other children.

Children cannot be kept in absolute ignorance about sexual matters because if the parents do not instruct them some one else will. Some one else always does.

The choice is then as to between correct, serious, sympathetic information, presenting sex as a tremendous fact of capital importance to the individual and the race, a great source of happiness and misery and, on the other hand, whispered gossip of the most fantastic type, dealt out by children, by ignorant or vicious adults, casting upon sexual phenomena and activities an obscene, romantically attractive light, leading to overindulgence, perversions, obsessions, etc.

Sexual information imparted by the ignorant or the vicious does not satisfy the child, does not stop his inquiries, and only causes him to seek more details, to probe the fascinating fiction he has heard, to build up around it the most dangerous form of romance.

Accurate information of a scientific type stops inquiries and day-dreams and vouchsafes to the child's mind the peace that comes with the securing of evidential facts, satisfactory to one's reason.

[68]

Mental rest is necessary to the child. The child's mind is so burdened with the thousand problems of adaptation and conduct, which confront a growing human being that the added pressure of sexual curiosity has been known in many cases to bring about neurotic symptoms.

Three children have been studied at close range by some of the greatest analysts. One boy, little Hans, studied by Freud and in whom sexual curiosity created an obsession which caused him to think of the male genitals in connection with almost every person or object he beheld; another boy, little Arpad, examined by Ferenczi and who, failing to secure information from human beings, addressed himself to the fowls in the henyard and identified himself with them; and finally, little Anna, treated by Jung, who in her search for a solution of the birth problem, propounded the most picturesque theories of life and death, lost all confidence in her mother and almost merged in a neurosis.

The case of the $3\frac{1}{2}$ year old Arpad, illustrates well the mental distortions which, at the time when children begin to develop a strong sexual curiosity, fear may cause in them, if connected with the subject of their eager inquiries.

Arpad and his parents went to spend a summer

in the country and stopped at a house which had a barn yard. Until then, Arpad's behaviour had been that of any normal, intelligent child of his age. He was interested in the various children's games and toys.

That summer, however, a complete change came over him. His toys were forsaken and he did not seek the company of other children. From early morning till he was sent to bed, he would spend all his hours in the poultry house, watching the chickens with tireless attention, imitating their clucking and their motions and, when forcibly removed, grew generally very indignant.

Even when led away from the fowl run, he did nothing but crow and cackle. He finally seemed to abandon words to use clucks, addressed people and answered their questions with sounds that imitated the cock's and hen's calls until his parents became quite concerned and feared he might loose his power of speech.

Arpad's attitude never changed during the summer. When his family took him back to town, he resumed human speech but could not be made to talk of anything but cocks, hens, chicks, sometimes of ducks and geese.

No toy appealed to him any more. He would all day long form little cocks and hens out of crumpled newspaper and offer them for sale to imaginary buyers. He then armed himself with some small object, called it a knife, went to the kitchen sink and declared that he was cutting the throat of his paper chickens. He imagined the animal bleeding and by various contortions mimicked strikingly its agony. Whenever the family purchased live chickens, he showed extreme excitement and his greatest joy was to attend the slaughtering of those fowl. He was however quite afraid of live cocks.

The parents plied him with many questions and always elicited from him the same story: once while playing in the chicken coop he wanted to micturate and a rooster pecked him painfully. The child was then two and a half years old.

Brought into Ferenczi's office, Arpad at once caught sight of a little bronze representing a mountain cock and asked for it. Given a pencil and paper he proceeded to draw a picture of a cock.

Mental examination proved impossible and Ferenczi had to confine his study to the mother's observations.

Early in the morning, Arpad would wake up the household with his lusty crowing. He sang continually but all the songs had to do with chickens.

He drew all day long pictures of birds with large beaks.

His parents yielded to necessity and bought him unbreakable toys representing chickens. They proved unsatisfactory as he could not cut off their necks. He would sometimes throw them into the oven, then take them out, clean them and caress them.

Several times he attempted to break a vase which had cocks painted on it. He often expressed a desire to put out the eyes of live or slaughtered chickens he saw in the house, and gave vent to other sadistic and also masochistic tendencies.

He identified himself and his family with barnyard fowl saying that his father was the rooster, his mother the hen, he himself a chicken and he once told a woman of the neighbourhood that when he grew old and became a rooster, he would marry her, her sister, his three cousins and the cook, and perhaps his mother too.

This remark was the key to the enigma of the child's conduct. Arpad had probably spied on his parents and the activities of the barnyard, the sexual activities of cocks and hens, the laying of eggs, the hatching of the little chicks had given him answers for all the riddles which his parents had refused to solve.

[72]

With a certain logic he had that summer given up the language of human beings who were, so to speak, silent to his questioning, and he had adopted that of the barnyard beasts who answered all his questions and illustrated for him all the processes of reproduction.

His cruelty toward chickens and his constant desire to cut off their necks was a natural reaction to his being pecked and to a fear of castration due to a foolish servant's threat.

A repetition of the same threat caused him to propound many questions as to the problem of death, angels and heaven. Later he began to occupy himself with religious thoughts. Old bearded beggars impressed him deeply and at the same time attracted and frightened him. Often after watching one of them he would let his head hang down and say: "Now I am a beggar chicken."

The animals who had satisfied his curiosity had also supplied him with a model with which to identify himself.

Very logically he had decided to cast in his lot with the knowing instead of the ignorant. His parents and other adults "did not know," the chickens "knew."

The little girl observed by Jung, Anna, was a healthy, intelligent, lively child of three, who had never been seriously sick and whose nerves seemed to be in excellent condition.

She once asked her grandmother whether she would become young again. Her grandmother explained to her that she would grow older and older and finally die and become an angel.

And then, little Anna asked, "Will you again become a baby?"

This was not the child's first attempt at solving the great problem of the origin of human life.

Her father had explained to her that children were brought by the stork; then some one else imparted to her the supplementary information that the stork picked them up in heaven where they were living as angels.

The remark made to her grandmother revealed the relatively enormous mental exertion, considering the child's age, to which Anna had submitted herself. Children are angels brought down by the stork; grandmother after death will go to heaven and become an angel; then probably she will be picked up some time by the stork and become a baby.

This solved more or less satisfactorily the problems of birth and death. Death became a picturesque experience of a romantic type devoid of any horror and holding out hopes of rejuvenation.

[74]

Very soon after, her mother became pregnant. Anna apparently did not notice the fact or, if she did, failed to mention it.

A few hours before the mother's delivery, Anna's father took the child on his knee and asked her: "What would you do if you should get a little brother tonight?" "I would kill it," Anna answered simply, without emotion, which in view of her theories of death and resurrection, implied merely that she would send the child back where it came from.

On the other hand, she undoubtedly had developed by that time her death-birth theory, for she asked her mother when admitted to her room, "What is going to happen now? Are you not going to die?" [1]

---

[1] Bleuler cites the case of a little girl three and a half years old who, after the coming of a baby in the household, also constructed a theory of life and death.

She was extremely interested in the baby and its nursing. When bitten once by a mosquito she was heard to remark that a little breast was growing on her, and she resented greatly the disappearance of the swelling as the bite healed.

One day her mother told her the story of the Ugly Duckling and she showed keen interest in it. She constantly asked to have the story repeated, especially that part of it in which the duck brings forth young ones. The wording of her request for the story reveals the problem which was on her mind: "Tell me about the *lady* and how the *children* come," although she knew that the tale dealt with a duck, not with a woman.

Asked once why she liked the story so well she said: "Because it gives me so much pleasure."

Sent to spend a few weeks with her grandmother while her mother was recuperating, Anna constantly reverted to questions concerning the stork theory. When she returned she appeared annoyed and suspicious. While not hostile to the baby, she would keep away from it and sit for hours under a table, mournful and dreamy, at times singing to herself little songs she improvised and in which the nurse seemed to play an important part.

At times, too, she would grow rebellious; she threatened to abandon her mother and to go to live with her grandmother. Once, finally, the result of her long cogitations revealed itself in an unexpected outburst.

"We are going into the garden," her mother said to her.

"Don't tell lies, Mamma," Anna answered.

"What are you thinking of? I always tell the truth," the mother said.

"No, Mamma, you are not telling the truth."

"You will see; come with me into the garden."

"What gives you pleasure?"

"The way in which the little children come out."

Immediately after she added:

"I dreamt that Suppenkaster (a character in a children's story) fell into the toilet."

Suppenkaster in the story becomes thinner and thinner and finally dies. *After death he grows again.*

This child's theory was not essentially different from that built by little Anna.

[76]

"And so it is really true? You were not lying?"

This amazing conversation had only one meaning. Her observations had convinced her that the death-and-birth-stork-and-angel theory was an imposition and that, consequently, both her father and mother were liars. As the idea of relativity is very undeveloped in the young, if her mother lied in one case, she was bound to lie in every case and a simple statement like "We are going into the garden" was only another of her mother's fabrications.

About that time, the Messina earthquake caused the child to develop an intense scientific curiosity based mainly on fear. She spent hours in her father's library looking for pictures of volcanoes and lava flowing out of the earth. Her questioning assumed a different aspect. She would ply her parents with questions like the following:

"Why is Sophie (her little sister) younger than I? Where was Freddie (the baby) before? What was he doing in heaven? Why didn't he come down sooner?"

Her parents, noticing her nervous eagerness, decided to tell her a part of the truth. Freddie, she was told, grew in the body of the mother as flowers develop out of a plant.

This occasioned more questions:

[77]

"How did Freddie come out? Since he cannot walk, did he crawl out? And is there a hole in the breast or did he come out of the mouth? Why don't babies come out of the nurse or the servant?"

One day, when her father was compelled by indisposition to remain in bed, Anna approached him with the inquiry:

"Have you a plant growing in you too?"

Her dreams showed a constant preoccupation with the birth problem and were offering solutions for them; Noah's ark with animals falling out of it, spring and summer days with all the flowers coming out.

A visit to a pregnant neighbour brought out a curious comparison between the woman's body and certain flowers and fruit. Then one day at the table, Anna took an orange announcing that she was going to swallow it, after which she would have a baby.

We must point out the remarkable similarity between the child's fancy and the various theories found in fairy tales and according to which pregnancy is produced by the eating of certain foods.

Thus Anna solved the problem of how children enter the mother's body. After which the rôle played by the father in the bringing forth of chil-

dren began to occupy her thoughts. Certain remarks she made seemed to imply that she had been
spying on her parents.

That manifestation of childlike curiosity often
has disastrous consequences. The child who has
watched the sexual act performed by his parents
and cannot by any means understand its meaning
may carry away the most horrifying impressions.

Some children are terrified and obsessed by what
seems to them a scene of violence. Some may develop frigidity or impotence later in life owing to
the disgust they experienced. Some may be
goaded into spying some more and waste much time
and energy keeping themselves awake and waiting
for a new opportunity. Some, identifying themselves with the overpowering father, develop strong
sadist, cruel traits, others, identifying themselves
with the mother, will on the contrary, be masochistic
perverts. Others will, owing to their ignorance of
anatomy and physiology, develop curious obsessive ideas of an analerotic type.

Little Anna had, therefore, reached a very critical stage at which definite action had become im-
perative.

Her father finally decided to satisfy her curiosity. Confronted one day with a demand for explanations as to who planted in her mother the seed

from which her little brother grew, he gave her the following answer suggested by Jung:

"The mother is like the soil of the garden, and the father like the gardener. The father plants in the mother the seed from which babies grow."

The explanation proved satisfactory and the little girl, after receiving confirmation of the truth which she suspected, that children come out the mother's genitals, ceased to cudgel her brain with the vexing problem which for two years had disturbed her so profoundly.

Little Arpad's and Little Anna's cases point out a practical solution for the problem of sexual enlightenment of children.

Explanations based upon botanical phenomena do not satisfy the children, their little minds unused to generalizations cannot draw from stories of pollen and seeds conclusions applicable to human beings. Parents must either become the sexual educators of their children or allow some one else to play that part. A teacher or the family physician and no one else, is qualified to undertake such a task.

The parents themselves, however, properly instructed by a competent person, would be the best persons to open their children's minds to such important facts. By denying them such knowledge,

[80]

they give to their children an impression of ignorance and expose themselves to the implied scorn which little Arpad revealed unconsciously by addressing himself to fowls. By telling lying stories they lose the confidence of their children and cause them to question every statement they may make later in life on vital subjects.

The revolt against the father's authority is certainly due in many cases to the hostility and jealousy which the boy feels against the man who monopolizes his mother's attentions, but in many cases too, the apparent stupidity and unreliability of the parents as a source of information on important matters, as exemplified by their dodging and fibbing about sex, is likely to exacerbate a boy's egotistical sense of superiority.

If parents wish to lead their children they must obviously be ahead of them. If parents appear either ignorant of certain facts known to many of the child's associates, or too bashful to discuss things which his little school chums or some shady characters with whom he may be in contact, discuss openly and without much embarrassment, the child can only draw one conclusion, that his parents are either lacking in knowledge or in courage, or hopelessly behind the times.

Parents often wonder why their children in

school and out of school generally follow the wrong leader. If a child is nice, modest, well behaved and soft spoken, he will get very little credit in school from his associates. He will not be taken as a model, and never will be a leader. The little Lord Fauntleroy has a miserable time of it in school and gets a lot of hazing.

The foul-mouthed urchin, on the other hand, who swears and knows obscene words and seems to lead a romantically indecent life out of school excites everybody's curiosity and his advice is taken on every occasion. He is supposed to know things.

Children are great egotists, whose main ambition is to become grown ups and to be treated as such. They wish to be taken seriously and resent being considered as mentally inferior beings.

The bad boy acts "like a man" and his "wisdom" and "knowledge" make it easy for him to assume the leadership of "the gang."

With a little more knowledge and less fear of certain words and facts, parents could retain their authority and save their children from many mistakes committed while emulating the bad boys.

The question of the sexual enlightenment of children goes much farther than the mere problem of telling children accurate facts about sex. It has an important bearing upon all the relations between parents and children.

BIBLIOGRAPHY

The analysis of Little Hans by Freud is not accessible to English readers. The cases of Little Arpad and Little Anna, however, are infinitely richer in their psychological applications and can be found in all their detail in S. Ferenczi's "Contributions to Psychoanalysis" (Badger) and Jung's lectures on "The Association Method," published by Clark University. The treatment accorded to children in the various epochs of history is well described in G. H. Payne's "The Child in Human Progress" (Putnam's).

The various problems of childhood are discussed thoroughly by H. V. H. Hellmuth, a woman physician, in "The Mental Life of the Child" (Nervous and Mental Disease Pub. Co.) and by William A. White, superintendent of St. Elizabeth Hospital for the Insane, Washington, D. C., in "The Mental Hygiene of Childhood" (Little, Brown), two books which should be read by every parent and educator. See also "The Problem of the Nervous Child" by Elida Evans (Dodd, Mead).

III. PROGRESS AND REGRESSIONS

CHAPTER I. THE NEGATIVE AND THE POSITIVE LIFE

The positive human being aims at a goal which is ahead, in time and space, and perhaps at a higher level than the one on which he presently stands. He makes plans for a future of useful activity, of beneficial endeavour and of social co-operation. He expects to encounter problems and to solve them in his own way, perhaps in a novel way.

The negative human being, on the contrary, seems fascinated by the past, seems to live in the past. He is constantly seeking some abnormal, unpleasant, painful form of regression, resorting to unsocial, selfish means, avoiding problems, and when he has to solve them himself, proving a slave to precedents.

Since all men should obviously be positive, why do so many lead a negative life? Why do so many regress instead of advancing? Why do so many destroy instead of being constructive?

Neurotics, perverts and criminals regress: neurotics ransack their past life for ready made solutions which, in the majority of cases, cannot be made to fit modified conditions; perverts seek sexual gratification in ways which are childish and imperfect; criminals revert to ethics of the primeval days, when each man or each beast, ignorant as yet of any form of solidarity, assaulted every other man or beast.

Regression is invariably due to some feeling of inferiority. Some people develop a weak heart. After which a rapid ascent up steep stairs, overindulgence in dancing, or a hearty meal may be followed by discomfort which makes the owner of the inferior organ keenly conscious of his inferiority. Some of us have capricious stomachs or fatigued eyes, bad teeth, a bald skull, thin arms, fat legs, lungs which are too sensitive to changes in the temperature, etc.

And most of us take those imperfections as granted. We do not worry over them, we reach some crompromise between life as we would lead it if we could and the life which our inferior organ allows us to lead; the man with a weak heart shuns dances and avoids excitement; the man with a poor digestion may select from the bill of fare a hundred dainties which demand no gastric strenuosity; the man with poor eyes picks out

[88]

books in large print; the thin person favours a fat-
tening diet; the obese one selects a diet likely to
bring him back to pleasant proportions; the bald
man avoids exposing his skull to icy blasts; the
person with decayed teeth uses a nut cracker. . . .

All of them, as long as they are normal, find
enough enjoyment in the long list of activities which
do not aggravate their condition; all of them come
to the conclusion that "it cannot be helped" and
let it go at that.

In certain cases the problem is more complicated.
Baldness or bad teeth or palpitations are obvious
facts and the discomfort they bring in their wake is
easily traced to its true source.

There are many organs, however, whose location
in our body is very vague to most of us, whose
names we do not even know, which are not painful
when diseased or deranged, and yet whose faulty
functioning may cause distressing symptoms.
Overactive adrenals, causing by their secretion of
adrenin, a constant sense of arterial tension, may
cause us to experience obscure feelings of discomfort which we express by saying: "I don't feel
right, I feel out of sorts, etc." The normal man
has himself examined carefully by a physician and
follows the treatment prescribed, and unless the
treatment seems to fail absolutely to relieve him,

goes about his business and does not pay too much attention to his condition.

The neurotic, on the contrary, dramatizes his inferiority, and instead of looking hopefully at all the opportunities which are open to him IN SPITE of that inferiority, dwells constantly and stubbornly upon the handicaps which it places on him, on the pleasures, advantages, privileges, which palpitations of the heart have removed from his reach, the attitudes his bald pate would spoil, etc.

In the case of unlocalized, obscure feelings of discomfort, he may become despondent, expect death or a lingering illness, lose his desire for life, let himself drift.

At times, a sense of inferiority is forced upon perfectly normal people by an environment which they have allowed to dominate them too completely.

Healthy young men and women may develop a deep sense of sin when they find themselves constantly reproved for the "impulsive" acts, the unrestrained enthusiasm, the outbursts of demonstrative affection which are natural to strong, full-blooded human beings.

In small communities, in puritanical circles, which are only too often dominated by oldish, sexually starved, narrow-minded old maids of both sexes, most manifestations of vitality are likely to be characterized as low, animal, bestial. Young women of an exuberant nature, who crave the perfectly legitimate excitement and the active life of an actress, of a concert artist, of an interpretative dancer, are the particular butt for such attacks.

Either they leave their environment in a rash way which not infrequently entails suffering or regrettable entanglements, or they allow their environment to indicate their conduct, they judge themselves as severely as their critics judge them, they co-operate with their critics in repressing normal cravings which soon proceed to seek an abnormal outlet in the form of hysteria, headaches, torturing states of anxiety.

Or they accept weakly their environment's estimate of their character with a discouraged "I am no good" as their justification and become a plague or a plaything for the world, drifting into promiscuity, prostitution or "insanity."

As neither normal nor abnormal people can carry happily through life a feeling of inferiority, they assume after a while a certain attitude which brings them consolation or compensation.

The best and most fruitful attitude in such cases is the following: In one respect I am inferior but in other respects, I am or can be superior.

The positive man striking that attitude will strive for some form of superiority: he may become an inventor of genius, a creator of new things, an artist, a writer. He may devise novel ways of curing his inferiority, of exercising the inferior organ (Adler has noticed that many people became chefs because they originally had a poor stomach and that many singers start singing as the best way of developing their inferior throat).

Accomplishment of some sort will restore the confidence which a feeling of inferiority may have weakened; it will compensate for the satisfactions which mere inferiority places beyond the inferior man's reach and offset the feeling that something is wrong somewhere in the organism. By accomplishment, I mean the kind of positive, creative activity which receives a measure, however small, of recognition.

Negative people and in certain cases, the originally positive people who go to extremes, may be more tortured by their attempts at compensation than they were by the inferiority for which they are attempting to compensate.

The world is acquainted with the many crazy inventors who are pestering their friends with some mechanical trifle they consider tremendous, with the cranks who would make the world an ideal place by banishing cigarette smoking, the uninspired poets, the undramatic playwrights, and too often, the true men of genius whose fame is to be a posthumous one.

Not a few merge into a deep melancholia on account of their failure to impress the world with the importance of their fad, not a few are aroused to acts of maniacal violence by the indifference with which their "discoveries" are received.

Another attitude which the inferior human being may adopt is expressed by the statement: Other people too are inferior.

This may be a basis for a healthy and normal compromise with life. I should not take my inferiority too tragically for many other people have a weak heart and yet enjoy life; many have imperfect features and yet have found love, etc. A realization of mankind's imperfections is a good antidote for the romantic view adopted by many sentimental beings and which in too many cases leads them to idealize strangers, to make gods and goddesses of people to whom distance lends many graces.

Such a realization may be very constructive in its results, for with it may go an intelligent sympathy for fellow sufferers, more tolerance, more patience, more kindness for other members of the social body, who are burdened with the same or similar handicaps.

That understanding is often a source of definite ego-satisfaction and the inferiority is often accepted gratefully on account of the mental superiority to which it leads. "Not until I was a sufferer from . . . did I understand, etc." is one statement frequently met with, and which is uttered with a certain amount of pardonable pride.

The negative type, on the other hand, the neurotic individual convinced of his inferiority, will not have any peace until he proves to himself and to others that ALL human beings are inferior, not only in ways similar to his but in many other respects.

His level will appear to him extremely low until he has dragged mankind down to the same level or even to a lower one. Without doing himself any appreciable good and without accomplishing anything positive, he destroys his environment's equilibrium and ultimately his own.

He begins a campaign of disparagement which impugns every statement, every act, every motive, aims at dwarfing every accomplishment, attributes sordid or unethical reasons to every form of activity that comes within his ken.

He casts reflections on other people's morals,

spreads vague rumours about their health, their disposition, their financial status. The gossip-monger enjoys a measure of power due to his reputation for having a sharp tongue; some, deceived by his spurious fearlessness, may respect him, some of his victims may fear him.

But there grows around him a more or less concealed hostility which he soon capitalizes in order to lend plausibility to his scorn and hatred of the world.

Scorn and hatred may soon lead him into introversion, that is, withdrawal from human society, from social groups, which he characterizes as too superficial, from crowds, which he denounces as vulgar, from friendly intercourse, which he presents as a waste of time.

The foundation is laid for the introversion of *dementia praecox* in which the patient gradually withdraws into himself paying no more attention to his environment, interested only in his own thoughts, staring at unseen things and in some cases assuming the prenatal position of the fetus in the mother's womb.

Another attitude which individuals may assume in order to compensate for a feeling of inferiority is the "sour grape" attitude. Within certain limits it is helpful. The man who fails to attain a certain object may console himself by letting his mind dwell on the advantages instead of on the unfortunate side of his failure. "That position would have been advantageous but it would have meant less freedom, etc." The jilted suitor may remember certain unpleasant traits of his sweetheart which might have made life with her a doubtful venture. The neurotic, on the other hand, proceeds to disparage all the goals which are beyond his reach. Unprepossessing bachelors of both sexes are very loud in their denunciation of the badness of men and women respectively. Ugly persons destined to be wall flowers criticize the dances at which they are not welcome and the low neck gowns which would expose their lack of charms. Not only do they deny vociferously their desire for "sour grapes" but they condemn all attempts on the part of others at reaching the goals which have eluded them. Negative in their life, they become teachers of negativism. They say "No" to life, because life said "No" to them and they avenge themselves by discouraging all those who, young and healthy, would say "Yes" to life.

A craving for safety is natural in all living things and constitutes one of the essential conditions of individual or group survival. The race which is not afraid of other, more aggressive races, which disregards the dangers accruing from epidemics and does not insure its future by permanent agencies of welfare, the individual who fails to stop, look and listen at crossings and never looks before he leaps, has an interesting but abbreviated career.

It is especially when our organism is not absolutely perfect that we must exercise very special care to offset that handicap. The man with a weak foot should not take chances and cross avenues in front of swiftly moving vehicles. The man with weak eyes should not jump until he has estimated very accurately the distance between starting and landing points; the man with weak kidneys should avoid strong beverages, etc.

Normal and inferior persons can indulge their craving for safety in perfectly positive ways, arriving at a compromise between what they would like to do and what they can safely do without injury to life and limb, without loss of money or of social prestige, etc. The positive person asks: "How can I safely do a certain thing?"

The abnormal neurotic person on the other hand will ask: "What shall I avoid in order to be safe?"

In other words the positive person stresses the accomplishment, the negative lays emphasis on safety.

Here again, instead of looking into the future, the

[97]

negative neurotic looks into the past for precedents. "How did I once find safety?"

This means, as usual, a regression to a younger
and younger stage, to one in which safety was as-
sured by the parents, guardians or teachers, who
solved all problems as soon as they arose, constantly
created precedents for conduct and made all planning for the future unnecessary. Thousands of
neurotics thus run back to father or mother in a
symbolic way.

We are all acquainted with the man who uses as a
criterion of his and other people's actions what "his
poor father" would have thought of them, with the
woman who does a certain thing because "it would
have made mother happy," and also with the men
and women who refrain from doing perfectly
simple, legitimate, harmless things because their
father or mother disapproved of them. Thousands
are Democrats or Republicans because of their
fathers' political affiliations and for no other conscious reason.

Such people are naturally hostile to every change,
be it in fashions or in government, because, very
naturally, there was nothing in their past which
constitutes a precedent for harem skirts or munic-
ipal ice houses, for cubism or original surgical
methods.

[98]

The feeling of strangeness experienced by many neurotics is easily explained as a regression to the past. Life goes on, but they either linger at one level or sink to a lower one and reality is to them a more and more puzzling phenomenon.

The old-fashioned type is often the product of a sense of inferiority, lack of adaptability and elasticity, low power of assimilation, coupled with an abnormal desire for safety.

This attitude very often assumes a sexual complexion which may deceive superficial observers.

The inferior male, who obscurely fears that he might not come up to the expectations of a sexual partner, disparages all women and seeks safety on the pedestal of his self-assumed masculine superiority. The inferior female pretends to scorn all males. The inferior husband surrounds his wife with varied protective devices which are ostensibly meant to protect her, and imply her inability to protect herself. He dictates what she may read, whom she may properly meet, what she should wear, in reality, isolating her as completely as possible from other more attractive and perhaps more virile males.

The inferior wife nags her husband into giving up "habits," friends, clubs, membership in associations likely to supply him with alibis; in brief,

[99]

she protects him from women more attractive than she is by constantly asserting her ownership of him and excluding from his circle of acquaintances all sources of possible temptation.

Inferior persons of both sexes only feel safe when the opposite sex has been humiliated. Men and women alike have contributed to the hostility between sexes as a consequence of which the masculine domination which is now gradually yielding to the onslaughts of feminists, implanted itself for many centuries.

And this leads us to a consideration of the will-to-power from its positive and negative sides.

The will-to-power is a normal striving of the living being for the natural result of regular, unhampered growth, physical and mental, of the perfect functioning of all the bodily agencies of acquisition, assimilation, metabolism and elimination: power.

Health and power are synonymous; power to resist death, power to do one's tasks without a feeling of exhaustion; power to join in all the world's activities; power for enjoyment; power to be used in emergencies. Every normal man or woman desires and seeks that form of power.

The will-to-power, on the other hand, becomes negative when the craving for it is synonymous with

[100]

a desire to destroy, not to create, to overpower others, not to be their equal in every respect.

Instead of the positive statement: I must be strong, the neurotic says, unconsciously: "I must appear as though I were strong."

Ferenczi cites the very striking case of a weak, neurotic clerk who, when submitted to some humiliation by his employer, went out to seek some male prostitute. Instead of being strong, manly, and either meeting the insult with proud rebuff or making himself more valuable and more worthy of respect, the poor neurotic spent some money, representing power, in order to subdue to his will and to humiliate some wretched man of the gutter.

And indeed, that psychology is not as rare as one might think; to many a neurotic, physical relations are symbolical of a humiliation of the woman; many a jealous neurotic has confessed to me that his worse torture was not the suspicion that his wife's affection was growing less but that some other man might subject her to his will even as he himself did.

Innumerable neurotic disturbances, epilepsy, sick headaches, dizziness, fainting spells, are expedients enabling the sick to indulge their will-to-power in a negative way. Instead of accumulating strength, they wear out the strength of those with whom they come in contact and who have to take care of them. Many an epileptic, facing defeat, "throws" a fit and thus gains an advantage he could not claim justly.

The woman with a sick headache silences the entire household; the dizzy person suffering from agoraphobia, requires an escort; the person who faints commands the services and the attention of all those present. None of those neurotic sufferers is conscious of that procedure but almost all of them confess naïvely some time or other to the pleasure vouchsafed them by the prompt succour offered them.

And in that naïve avowal there is concealed one more egotistical satisfaction: "You see how appreciative I am. . . ." This is one form of unconscious hypocrisy very noticeable in people with a weak heart. They promptly exploit the popular superstition which makes the heart the centre of all the tender emotions and boast of their sensitiveness which naturally makes them more sympathetic and places a new duty upon those whom they unconsciously victimize.

Self-knowledge as acquired through analysis or self-analysis, is the only protection against a negative orientation, against an attitude which is disastrous to the sufferer and his environment. For

[102]

while the neurotic derives infinite unconscious satisfaction from his abnormality he consciously goes through the tortures of hell. His spurious superiority and power do not satisfy him consciously. And this is one of the reasons why he is so easily aroused, so vituperative and insulting in disputes. From this he again derives a certain superiority. People are afraid of discussing any subject with a neurotic and oftentimes yield point after point in order to avoid unpleasantness.

The neurotic obscurely feels that his arguments are not valid, that his position is untenable, that his evidence could not stand any test and his anger at his own powerlessness is projected on those who cross-examine him. He is like a man who has been hypnotized and unconsciously invents very plausible reasons for proving that he did of his free will what the hypnotist commanded him to do.

Insight into our unconscious, like the gradual and detailed explanations of the hypnotist to his subject, allows both neurotic and medium to realize that they were subjected for a while to an abnormal influence and that to a certain extent "they were not themselves."

The problem to solve constantly in human conduct is: "Am I myself, is it I myself who am speaking and acting or is it my unconscious self,

[103]

attempting to follow the line of least resistance, leading me toward regression instead of progress, toward the past instead of toward the future?"

Conduct based upon that system alone might not be perfectly normal. Introversion and extroversion, that is the fixation of our attention upon ourselves or upon exterior objects, can both be normal and abnormal. Extreme introversion, the detachment of our interest from the entire world and its fixation on ourselves alone means absolute negativism; extreme extroversion, the constant chasing of a new butterfly, exaggerated interest in every passing fad or detail of life, means the squandering of our resources, mental and physical, on a hundred goals none of which is ever reached.

He who attempts too many things is almost as unproductive as he who withdraws from reality.

Our reactions to stimulus words and our dreams alone can give us a clear picture of our orientation. Introversion and extroversion are easily determined by even a superficial examination of the first and our dreams reveal to us accurately what our unconscious is trying to make us do.

The Aschner test described on page 40 is a simple way of confirming the diagnosis.

He whose reactions reveal him as extremely self-

centred and introverted should be on his guard
against that tendency and force himself to adopt
attitudes which will lead to fewer conflicts with his
environment.

The overmodest person burdened with a feeling
of inferiority can go through a systematic training
of ego-building and personality development.

In other words, those who have been deceived
by their unconscious and who know to what extent
the deception has gone, may discount their first impressions and withhold final judgment until they
have ascertained whether their conscious I or their
unconscious I is responsible for that first impression and is dictating their judgment.

We must now and then go through the process
which the Catholics call examination of conscience
and submit our attitudes to a test based upon the
following five propositions:

A tendency to constantly disparage is negative
and should put ourselves on our guard.

Desire for power that exalts us at the expense of
others is also negative.

The constant search for precedents is negative.

In brief, whatever enables us to harmonize with
our environment and to help it toward its goal is
positive.

[105]

Whatever creates disharmony between ourselves and our environment and retards its onward march is negative.

BIBLIOGRAPHY

For a study of the neurotic temperament consult William A. White's "Elements of Character Formation" and "Principles of Mental Hygiene," both published by Macmillan. "Human Motives," by J. J. Putnam, is a very simple presentation of the hidden forces which compel us to act abnormally at times.

The deepest and most searching analysis of the neurotic's mental workings will be found in A. Adler's "The Neurotic Constitution" (Moffat, Yard) which requires very careful reading, for it presupposes a certain knowledge of analytic methods and has been translated in rather heavy style.

CHAPTER II. SPEECH AND MEMORY DE-FECTS

The neurotic type in its negative attitude to life refuses to face unpleasant facts.   It adopts the ostrich's tactics and buries its head in the sand.   The most efficient way to flee from an unpleasant reality is not to know any longer that it was once perceived. Oblivion is the simplest way to rid oneself of an unpleasant fact.   If it cannot be entirely forgotten, avoiding to mention it is the next best negative expedient.   Loss of memory, partial or complete, obliterates a part of our biography which we lack courage to acknowledge as our own.   Aphasia, aphonia or stammering withhold conveniently statements which our unconscious considers damaging.

A German woman of fifty who at the beginning of the war had been especially loud in her progermanism and had thereby caused her family and relatives a great deal of annoyance, was absolutely prostrated when her son, a naturalized citizen, was drafted.   A panicky fear seized her lest her indiscrete utterances might bring punishment upon her beloved boy's head.

[107]

The night when he left for camp, she became strangely silent and the next morning she was absolutely disoriented, being unable to recognize any member of her family or her environment.

Her memory for everything which had occurred since August, 1914, was entirely gone; she could speak only with great difficulty and for a while her vocal cords lost all resonance; she regained to a certain extent her powers of speech when expressing herself in English but she was absolutely unable to make herself heard when she talked German.

On the other hand, her memory of events preceding the world catastrophe was absolutely unimpaired. While she never joined a conversation or addressed any one first she would very often supply with astounding accuracy facts or dates needed by those conversing in her presence. All the facts of her biography and of that of her children antedating 1914 were perfectly clear and well remembered, but when asked their age, she gave the age they had reached in August, 1914.

Here is a case then in which partial amnesia and partial aphasia proved a negative asset to the neurotic. The war which brought her much misfortune was forgotten. The voice which had carried to hostile ears many indiscrete statements was muted and the language which at a time none could
[108]

speak in public without being eyed suspiciously or ostracised, failed to make her vocal cords vibrate.

A stammerer engaged in scientific research never had any difficulty in mentioning a certain chemical whose methods of production he was trying hard to improve. One day, however, a fellow laboratory worker forestalled him in finding a more efficient device. At the next appointment, the stammerer was almost unable to tell me of the occurrence and could not for several minutes pronounce clearly the name of the chemical in question. His unconscious egotism was bent on withholding from me information of a humiliating character. As soon as the neurotic expedient became obvious to him, his impediment disappeared.

A woman compelled in self-defence to tell her husband a very complicated story lacking in plausibility, began to stammer whenever a word in her conversation seemed to be unconsciously associated with the compromising incident. A full confession in my office relieved the tension and the "watchful technique" did the rest.

A study of all cases of memory and speech disturbances will soon convince the observer that our memory does not retain or lose words and facts indiscriminately.

Stammerers do not stammer indiscriminately.

There always is an absurd unconscious reason, neurotically logical, which causes us to forget a word, a fact, a duty, a figure, or to lose partly or completely our powers of speech.

We may forget anything which has an unpleasant unconscious connotation, we may stammer on any word which has an unpleasant association or be totally unable to pronounce it.

Hence the usual methods for improving the memory are psychologically absurd.

We may memorize long lists of words or sentences, poems and orations and yet at the crucial moment the right word may be withheld because some unconscious complex makes it impossible for us to utter it.

Mnemotechnic methods which seek to create new and at times illogical and absurd associations of the "clang" type or of the pun type are better. They grant unconsciously what the analysts claim, that the associations conjured up by a word may be of such a nature that the word cannot be uttered and they seek to replace a natural and unconscious association by an unnatural and conscious one.

This involves however a gigantic amount of exertion and the results of this procedure cannot be permanent.

The removal of the complexes which hold words

[110]

down is the only scientific method for "improving" one's memory. Psychoanalysis does not, however, "improve" one's memory; it disintegrates the elements which impair our memory.

Our memory is simply the faculty our autonomic nerves have of making use, in an emergency, of impressions received in the course of our bringing up. When some fear-impression causes the safety division of the autonomic system to repress the natural activities of the other divisions, the words are, if the repression is complete, entirely forgotten, or if the repression is less complete, remembered but unpronounceable and, if the repression fails, stammered on more or less painfully.

The various cures suggested for stammering have never cured any one permanently.

Any stammerer can be trained to read without any difficulty lists of disconnected words and sentences of varying length. Any stammerer can be trained to sing without stammering.

This means that the words he studies lose gradually their present, unconscious associations and become mere sounds. As soon, however, as those words are grouped differently and acquire anew their unconscious associations, the stammerer once more becomes tongue-tied.

Making the sufferer change the pitch of his voice,

[111]

one popular method of treating stammerers, is just as inefficient. Called upon to single out one word and to treat it as a "vehicle" for sound, not for thought, the stammerer no longer feels any embarrassment. The embarrassment returns, however, when the stammerer has to speak in a natural, even tone of voice.

Experiments show that fixation of the reading glance on one word only at a time, helps the stammerer, for it accomplishes more simply the same purpose as a change of pitch. It disconnects each word from its context and hence rids it of its associations.

This is, however, little more than an expedient and does not go to the root of the matter.

Nothing avails except to free the subject from the unconscious complexes withholding the words on which he stammers.

The stammerer who gains insight into the mechanism of his disability, who realizes not only that every bothersome word, sound or even letter, is fraught with an unpleasant connotation, but, furthermore, that his stammering is a valuable negative asset for him, will gradually acquire perfect fluency of speech.

One stammerer I treated came to realize that his stammering enabled him to dominate his environ-

[112]

ment, as his mother and sister had to do all his shopping, receive and send all his telephone messages; he could keep his employer waiting for explanations, he could delay his answers and modify their wording (hereby satisfying his safety cravings). While he could pronounce without difficulty the name of any woman he was acquainted with, he could seldom pronounce men's names, especially when those men wielded some authority over him.

The usual memory and speech methods are based on the assumption that certain people are born with a poor memory or a "heavy tongue." Psychoanalysis assumes that all human beings are born with probably the same average ability but that in the course of their bringing up some of that average ability has been handicapped by complexes and cannot manifest itself freely. Instead of developing memory or fluency, psychoanalysis busies itself with the removal of the complexes which disable the patient.

This precludes the relapses which are so frequent and so discouraging in the treatment of amnesia, aphasia and stammering by the old fashioned methods.

BIBLIOGRAPHY

Very little has been published on stammering from the psychoanalytic point of view. See "Stammering as a Psychoneurosis" by Isador H. Coriat, *Journal of Abnormal Psychology,* Vol. IX, No. 6, and "Stammering as a Psychoneurosis and Its Treatment by Psychoanalysis" by M. D. Eder, Int. Med. Congress, Section of Psychiatry. Tr. XVII. See also A. Appelt: "Stammering and Its Permanent Cure." 1912.

CHAPTER III. SCAPEGOATS

Ever since man appeared on the earth he has felt the necessity of scapegoats. Frazer's monumental work "The Golden Bough" reveals thousands of obvious or subtle attempts on the part of mankind to saddle the responsibility for individual or group shortcomings on some unwilling or willing sacrificial victim, beast, man or god.

The Greek drama blamed fate, the Middle Ages the devil; one civilization sacrificed a goat whose death wiped off the sins of men; in another civilization, Jesus died to save mankind.

In our days, we no longer accuse the devil of causing our failures. "Popular science" spread thinly by Sunday newspapers and club lectures, supplies the masses with new impressive scapegoats.

"Racial traits," "inbreeding," "heredity," "environment," have been in a most hypocritical way substituted for the goat of old.

The pagan who sinned and, afraid of the impending reckoning, killed a goat in order to mollify some heavenly policeman, did not deny his

guilt. The modern "sinner" who seeks excuses for
his brutality or his lewdness in his heredity or his
environment, is guilty of a much more complete
flight from reality.

The pagan admitted that sinning was pleasant but
could not be indulged in unless there was one
more goat to be offered to the gods. The
modern sinner is consciously in fear of sin, but
unconsciously preparing his escape by heaping
up guilt upon vague biological processes which he
does not understand.

The pagan said: "I did not repress certain
cravings and I am willing to pay the price." The
modern sinner on the other hand says: "I could
not repress certain cravings, because my ancestry,
my bringing up or my environment have made it
impossible for me to suppress such cravings."

If the modern sinner has a conscience, such a
disclaimer of guilt may be perfectly honest and
straightforward and constitute for the person making it a great danger.

The hypocrite who exploits heredity and other
scapegoats as a convenient explanation for the
gratification of his own cravings is probably safe.
The ethically-minded person who believes that his
heredity or some other biological factor has unfitted him to repress unsocial, inadmissible crav-
[116]

ings may undergo very torturing "soul struggles" and be defeated in life's battle.

Physical heredity cannot be denied and Mendel's experiments prove that it is ruled by absolute mathematical laws. Not only do we observe in nature that certain characteristics of the parents are reproduced in an invariable proportion of the off-spring, but we can, before crossing certain animal or vegetable species, predict accurately how many of the offspring will present certain characters and how many will not present such characters.

This is as far as heredity goes. The transmission of mental characteristics is probably due to what Freud calls pseudo-heredity, that is to the influence wielded on the child by its environment, that environment consisting chiefly of the parents for the first years of the child's life.

Biologists generally agree that while inherited characters or congenital characters cannot be modified, acquired characters can be caused to disappear in later life.

Those who consider themselves as "burdened with a bad heredity" should ponder that fact. They should remember that even a weak or defective organ, stomach or lungs, may be, not inherited from the parents, but acquired under the same unfavourable circumstances which caused that inferiority to establish itself in their parents' organism.

A changed environment, proper exercise and plenty of food have been known, together with imitation of the proper model, to modify entirely the physical appearance of various races.

I have mentioned elsewhere that the so-called hereditary instincts can be absolutely "removed" by the influence of the environment.

When a messenger pigeon refuses to mate with its kind if hatched by a ring dove and then will only mate with ring doves, we must come to the conclusion that training is stronger than instinct.

When we observe that a change in temperature either shortens or prolongs the average life of a certain species or creates a different species, we must also conclude that environment is stronger than heredity.

Eggs from the same butterfly or puppae of the same species will give entirely different species at different temperatures.

The number of "hereditary characters" is decreasing year after year as scientists become more thorough in their observations and include in their statistics a growing number of factors.

It was admitted for centuries that some inherited

instinct caused fishes to rise to the surface of the waters at night and to go down to the bottom at dawn.

We know now that heredity has nothing to do with that phenomenon.

The presence of carbonic acid in water causes all aquatic animals to direct themselves toward the source of light. At night the waters of pools and rivers become charged with carbonic acid as the green aquatic plants cannot absorb that gas in the dark. Fishes and other organisms are affected by that excess of carbonic acid and are compelled to rise to the surface where the light, however feeble, is stronger than at the bottom.

In the morning, the supply of acid decreases rapidly and all the organisms regain their freedom and can seek safety in the deeper strata of the water.

By liberating large quantities of carbonic acid in the water during the day, one can compel all the aquatic organisms to rise to the surface, and by directing at night a strong light on the waters, which facilitates the absorption of carbonic acid by green plants, one can, on the contrary, cause the fishes to remain at the bottom.

It is not improbable that in a few years, many

[119]

obscure facts attributed to heredity or to instincts will be traced to physical or chemical phenomena which can be PRODUCED or REMOVED at will.

A French scientist, Pouchet, has noticed that certain fishes reproduce the colour or pattern of the aquarium in which they are kept PROVIDED THEY CAN SEE IT. Blind fishes of the same species, kept in the same aquarium, retain the whitish or greyish colour they had when they first came out of the egg. The so-called protective colouring of certain animals, the seasonal changes observed in the plumage of the ptarmigan, may not be more than mere unconscious imitation of the environment, devoid of any purpose. A very illuminating case of what we might call metachemistry.

Insanity, feeble-mindedness or criminality are not inherited characters. They are often acquired through either imitation or suggestion or both.

The insane and the criminal solve their problems by following the line of least resistance and least effort. The children they bring up are likely, unless some healthier influence is exerted on them, to solve their problems in the same way, the only way which observation has made thoroughly familiar to them.

Auto-suggestion and involuntary suggestion by
[120]

others play a powerful part in the acquisition of criminal or neurotic traits. In a crisis, the individual weakened by his superstitious belief in heredity, may either commit a crime or merge into a neurosis because his father, mother or grandfather established such a precedent. .

That precedent may not be more than a legend perpetuated by inaccurate, stupid or gossipy relatives.

A man guilty of some act of brutality is easily catalogued in family archives as a man of criminal instincts. A man of rather morose disposition very often has his trouble diagnosed by amateur psychiatrists in his family circle as melancholia.

A romantic legend may form after his death around his actual biography and invest some detail of behaviour, which on one occasion impressed the beholders, with the dignity of a life-long habit or of a serious mental disturbance.

The stupid parent who vents his anger on his offspring by making remarks such as "You are as crazy as your father (mother, uncle, aunt)," "You will end in jail as your uncle did," may start a train of suggestive thought which is highly dangerous.

I have known personally three brothers who were

brought up by an exceptionally idiotic mother and who on several occasions had themselves committed to an insane asylum when they lost their money or their jobs. None of them succeeded in remaining "insane" for any length of time, although all of them repeated constantly that they were "going crazy like their father." Inquiry showed that their father, who died when they were very young, had several fits of blues coinciding with slumps in the family's finances but never showed at any time any "insane" traits.

Men and women have been known to reproduce in their behaviour certain habits bad or good of their grandparents. Investigation showed in many of them, and would probably have shown in every one of them, that they were obsessed by the old belief that genius or vice, etc., "skips a generation."

"Racial psychology," a limited form of "mental" heredity, is, like heredity proper, a weapon directed against our enemies and a scapegoat for our own sins. To the honest psychologist, so-called racial traits amount merely to different sets of bad manners tolerated or encouraged in one community, discouraged and held shameful in other communities owing to reasons of temperature, climate, food supply, etc.

The unconscious make-up of all races, however,

is the same the world over as a careful analysis of all folk traditions, legends, religions, superstitions, ritual, neurotic psychology, etc., proves abundantly. It is as silly to expect a certain form of behaviour from one individual because he is a Jew or an Irishman as it would be for a Jew or an Irishman to excuse a certain form of behaviour of his on the plea that his antecedents determined certain psychological processes.

Inbreeding is another cause for worry which neurotics are likely to seize upon as a conscious screen for their unconscious strivings to escape reality.

There is absolutely no evidence of a scientific nature that the marriage of blood relations is productive of insanity or feeble-mindedness in the offspring.

But there are good reasons to suspect that feeble-mindedness leads to unions between blood relations and in many cases to incestuous unions. Parent fixation being stronger in neurotics than in normal individuals, the family complex is bound to attract related neurotics to each other. The result is that the children whom they procreate may be born normal but are brought up by their neurotic parents to adopt neurotic forms of action and thought.

Goddard, who has made exhaustive studies of

[123]

feeble-mindedness, has reached the conclusion that the feeble-minded are constantly thrown together, congregate in certain places and intermarry more than normal individuals.

That each neurotic family trains its children to one peculiar form of abnormal behaviour is well illustrated by the history of the sinister Juke family propagated by incestuous descendance: all the descendants of Ada were criminals, the descendants of Belle, exhibitionists or rapists, the descendants of Effie, beggars.

As against the tragic results of inbreeding among the inferior, we may remind the reader of the remarkable results of inbreeding among individuals of superior stock.

In Athens and her suburban communities between 530 and 430 B. C., that is during the heyday of Hellenic brilliancy, there was a small population from which came about fifteen of the most remarkable geniuses the world has ever known.

Inbreeding was the custom, marriage with half-sisters being lawful, and unions with aliens being discouraged.

The decline of the Hellenic civilization was not brought about by any racial decay but by the overwhelming pressure of primitive races of a more savage type invading a highly cultured region much as the desert sand gradually invaded the centres of culture of Mesopotamia and North Africa.

Some of the most wonderful specimens of agricultural products or animal breeds have been obtained through continual inbreeding. It is not therefore inbreeding which influences the mental quality, nor even the fact that one of the parents or both are neurotically inclined, but the fact that children are trained in a neurotic way.

Re-education, however, mental or physical, is fortunately a possibility which should never be overlooked.

We are born with general physical tendencies, that is, we reproduce closely the general type of the human variety to which we belong. We receive the bony, muscular and nervous structure of what will, according to the pains we take, become a statue or a scarecrow.

Imitation is mostly unconscious and a negative way of dealing with problems. Our parents are the first models presented to us by nature while we are casting about for some one to imitate. But they need not remain the only models from which we shall shape our statue.

Our parents may have fleshless limbs and poor lungs. But we can go to a gynasium, run around the track, lift weights, breathe fresh air, at least

[125]

all night long, regulate our diet scientifically, walk to and from work.

Our parents may be abnormal mentally, but libraries, lecture halls and meeting places will bring us into contact with active men and women who are normal and whom we can imitate, dispelling thereby the mental ghosts who thrive in the home atmosphere.

Animals are creatures of their environment and according to whether that environment is favourable or unfavourable, they die out or survive. Man is the creator of his environment and can change his surroundings at will.

Most of our heredity is a pseudo-heredity which, being simply the shaping influence of our environment, can be defeated as soon as we realize that it is not working for our welfare.

One question every one of us must ask himself frequently is: "Am I myself, or am I imitating some one and if I am imitating some one, am I following the line of least resistance?"

Another question is: "Do I believe in a certain thing or have I accepted this belief at some one's suggestion, and if so, what necessary task am I trying to shirk?"

One of Kempf's patients let her parents bring her up as a perfectly irresponsible woman and later, when that irresponsibility made her married life very unpleasant, instead of re-educating herself and solving her problems in a positive, constructive way, she accepted her relatives' dictum that "she was crazy," and became "crazy."

Kempf re-educated her; after becoming herself, she threw off the yoke of suggestion imposed upon her by silly relatives.

The day when the combined power of imitation and suggestion is realized, the knowledge of our abnormal ascendance will not trouble us. Instead of discouraging us and of causing us to say neurotically: "What can I do against such odds?" we shall study carefully the ways in which our progenitors or parents deviated from the normal standard and consciously train ourselves to avoid their physical and mental errors.

Heredity shall cease to be a menace and shall become in certain cases a warning and a guide.

When insight has delivered us from the absurd belief in fate, in the devil or some other overpowering metaphysical force which shall crush us and compel us to do what unconsciously we are craving to do, we shall be better off for an accurate knowledge of our so-called hereditary handicaps. We shall not allow ourselves to use them neurotically as scapegoats.

BIBLIOGRAPHY

William White's "Mechanisms of Character Formation" will enable the average reader to complete a picture which, owing to lack of space, had to remain rather sketchy. Advanced students should read the fourth part of J. G. Frazer's "Golden Bough" entitled "The Scapegoat" in order to fathom the psychology which has made scapegoats necessary.

The latest data on heredity can be found in two extremely technical volumes published under the auspices of the Rockefeller Institute, East and Jones "Inbreeding and Outbreeding" (Lippincott) and T. H. Morgan "The Physical Basis of Heredity" (Lippincott).

CHAPTER IV. DUAL PERSONALITIES

Every human being has two personalities: an archaic, primitive, childlike, unadapted personality, and a modern, sophisticated, adult, and, to all appearances, adapted personality.

Civilization and education have superimposed the second over the first or rather built over the first a thin crust of manners which does not permit its sharp angles to protrude.

When the operation of walling in the archaic personality is performed in a bungling way some of its sharp points have a tendency to crop out and when civilization tries to force back all those sharp points by exerting on the thin crust a pressure which it cannot bear, the archaic personality breaks through entirely and for a certain period of time refuses to be buried again.

Psychiatrists of the old school were extremely puzzled by cases of double personality and some spoke of dissociation of the brain, of two separate brains, of wrong associations of neurons or cell groups, etc.

To the psychoanalyst, a case of double personality is not any more mysterious than the simplest of our day or night dreams.

It is a neurosis which offers to the subject a means of escape from reality, which enables him to regress to a mode of life in which some or all of his responsibilities are removed, and which in no essential detail is different from the various forms of "insanity" for which psychiatrists have devised impressive and meaningless designations.

A brief review of the best known cases of double personality will help me to make my point clear.

The Rev. Ansel Bourne was a hard working clergyman of excellent character and reputation, enjoying the confidence of all his associates. His health was good and his muscular strength and endurance normal. Since childhood he had been subject to fits of "blues," and became easily depressed.

One day he drew $500 from a bank in Providence, boarded a Pawtucket car and disappeared for two months. Then his nephew in Providence received a telegram saying that a man claiming to be Rev. Ansel Bourne was in Norristown, Pa., acting strangely.

The man was not acting strangely, but very normally. He was in reality the Rev. Ansel

[130]

Bourne, who suddenly had found himself in a strange town and in a small fruit store.

Six weeks before his awakening, Bourne had gone to Norristown, rented a small store, stocked it with candy and fruit and had been doing business as A. Brown, living in the back of his shop where he cooked his own meals. His manners never attracted any one's attention. He went regularly to church, and once, at a prayer meeting, made a rather good address.

When the awakening came and he regained his former personality, he was very weak and had lost over twenty pounds in weight.

William James examined him and induced him to submit to hypnotism. In hypnosis the Brown personality came to the fore with surprising readiness and with such insistence that the subject could not remember any of the facts of his life as Ansel Bourne.

Brown didn't even "know" Ansel Bourne and repeated constantly that he felt "hedged in at both ends." He could not remember any of the incidents preceding the ride to Pawtucket, nor any of those following his awakening in Norristown. The only explanation he gave for his escapade was that "there was trouble back there" and "he wanted rest."

In this case the first personality did not know the second, nor did the second know the first.

In other cases one of the personalities was acquainted with the other, or both knew each other and in one case there was a distinct feeling of scorn and hatred, in the other a deep friendship manifested by both personalities for each other.

Miss Beauchamp, studied by Morton Prince, was a serious minded person, fond of books and study, very idealistic, "with a morbid New England conscientiousness" and a great deal of pride and reserve, very unwilling to expose herself or her life to any one's scrutiny.

One day "owing to some nervous excitement" she became an entirely different personality. She called herself Sally, a creature full of fun, unable to take anything seriously, scorning books and churchgoing, eager for all forms of amusement, lacking all the educational accomplishments of Miss Beauchamp, such as a knowledge of foreign languages and stenography.

Miss Beauchamp was a neurasthenic, Sally was always well, never fatigued and never seemed to suffer pain.

During the first year, Miss Beauchamp and Sally constantly alternated with one another. Whenever Miss Beauchamp felt tired or upset, Sally used to

[132]

appear, sometimes for a few minutes, sometimes for several hours. Later, Sally's appearances lasted several days at a time.

Miss Beauchamp never knew Sally, but Sally knew everything about Miss Beauchamp. Furthermore Sally hated her and said so very frankly.

She went as far as playing tricks on her to annoy her. She would mail to Miss Beauchamp a box full of spiders and snakes, she would ride to the end of a trolley line without return carfare and oblige her to walk miles or beg rides from passing wagons; she would unravel her knitting, she wrote her annoying letters, etc.

Alma Z., observed for ten years by Dr. Osgood Mason, had been in robust health until her 18th year, when "owing to overwork at school," she underwent a curious change. She had been until then an educated, thoughtful, dignified, feminine type. She suddenly became a cheerful, sprightly, childish person, ungrammatical, and using a peculiarly limited vocabulary.

She called herself Twoey and referred to her first personality as No. 1. Twoey would at first only remain a few hours but later her stay was prolonged to several days.

While "1" and "2" were apparently in every respect separate and distinct personalities, each took up life and its occupations where the other had left off.

Twoey knew "No. 1" well and "No. 1" became acquainted with Twoey through the descriptions given her by others.

The two personalities became great friends. Twoey admired "No. 1" for her superior knowledge, her patience in suffering and the lovely qualities which she recognized and she willingly took her place to give her rest.

"No. 1" also became fond of Twoey on account of the loving care she bestowed upon her and her affairs and for her witty sayings which she greatly enjoyed.

As Alma Z.'s health improved, Twoey's visits became scarce, and only coincided with conditions of extreme fatigue or mental excitement.

Then Alma married and became an excellent wife and an efficient mistress of the household.

One night, however, Twoey re-appeared but merely to announce that she was to disappear and that another personality, "The Boy," would take her place. The Boy submitted to all the duties which Alma had to discharge but when questioned persisted in declaring her male and youthful character. Alma knew Latin, mathematics, and philosophy, she had memorized entire poems by

Tennyson, Browning and Scott. The Boy was absolutely ignorant, although he had an intelligent grasp of affairs and manifested a keen enjoyment of theatrical and musical performances.

One evening at a concert in the Metropolitan Opera House, the Boy suddenly disappeared and Alma returned for a few minutes, but Alma soon closed her eyes and assumed the harsher, more masculine countenance of her boyish personality.

The Boy knew Twoey and "No. 1" and liked both of them. Like Twoey he expressed a constant desire that "No. 1" should get well and not need him any more.

Ansel Bourne had regressed to a lower intellectual level, but remained on an adult level. Miss Beauchamp and Alma Z. regressed to childhood. In the case of Mary Reynolds, we will observe a regression to infancy and in that of the Rev. Thomas Carson Hanna, to the condition of the newborn.

Mary Reynolds, treated by Dr. S. Weir Mitchell, was a shy, morose, melancholy woman. She had suffered frequently from convulsions, loss of consciousness, loss of sight and hearing.

After having been greatly weakened by a severe attack, she fell into a deep sleep from which she could not at first be aroused.

On awaking she was found to have lost all her

former knowledge, to be unable to recognize her environment or any of her friends.

She still knew how to eat, drink and walk, but she could neither speak nor understand spoken words. She was an infant, mumbling disconnected words. In her second state she was gay, lively and playful.

The transition from "1" to "2" always took place at night, that from "2" to "1" during the day time.

No case has been more completely described than that of Rev. Thomas Carson Hanna, treated by Dr. Boris Sidis and Dr. S. P. Goodhart.

Rev. Hanna had never suffered from any illness up to his twenty-fourth year when the slight accident, following which his personality changed, took place.

He was a versatile man, endowed with not only intellectual, but mechanical ability, showing artistic taste in many directions; he had a strong will and perfect self-control. He was not demonstrative in his affections and was influenced more easily by reason than by emotion.

One evening, returning home in his carriage, he lost his footing while alighting, fell head foremost and remained unconscious for two hours. When he regained his consciousness he had become as helpless as a newborn infant. He could neither

[136]

speak nor understand what was said to him. He did not know how to control his voluntary muscles, he could not walk. He had no conception of distance or time.

When food was offered to him he did not understand the purpose of it; nor, when it was placed in his mouth, did he know how to masticate and swallow it. It was only when food was forced upon him and thrust far back into the pharynx and reflex swallowing movements excited, that he realized the purpose of food and learned the way of taking it.

Like an infant, he satisfied his natural needs without regard to time or place. Like an infant, he began to learn a few words by imitating definite articulate sounds made in connection with certain objects. The first word he learnt was "apple" which to him meant all kinds of food.

His intelligence, however, was that of an adult. His memory was excellent. A word once heard seemed indelibly impressed on his mind and he never again forgot it.

Like an infant, he was trying to grasp things beyond his reach, such as a tree he saw out of the window. Like an infant, he did not at first discriminate between his motions and those of other people. Nor did he analyse complicated objects into their component parts; a man, a man on a bicycle, and a man sitting in a buggy were to him three different kinds of men. Life and motion were at first synonymous to him.

He gradually learnt to speak, to walk, to sing and to play instruments but he only knew the things he had studied since his change of personality had taken place. Everything and everybody he had known previous to that time was absolutely forgotten. Once, the reading aloud to him of a Hebrew passage with which he was familiar brought to consciousness a flow of Hebrew quotations which he, however, did not understand.

Seven weeks after the accident, about three o'clock in the morning, he awoke to find himself in a strange house in New York City. He demanded explanations from his brother who was sharing his room.

When Dr. Goodhart, at whose house he was staying, came into the room he took him for a perfect stranger.

All memory of the events intervening between April 15 at seven o'clock in the evening and June 8 in the early morning had faded.

In fact he resumed his conscious life at the very hour of the day when he had sunk into unconsciousness and insisted that it must be evening. On the other hand, he recounted as a part of his actual life some of the incidents of which he had been dreaming in hypnoidic states of his second personality.

On June 9 about 4 P. M. he fell asleep and when he awoke he had relapsed into his second personality. This time, however, he merely continued the life he had led before in that state and carried on the memories of it. He had not regressed further than that.

He gained much insight into his condition and, when told by his brother of his various changes of personality, appeared greatly depressed. He asked anxiously whether there would not be a third state in which he would not remember either his normal or his second personalities.

All sorts of stimulation were resorted to, from chemicals to a variety performance, in order to arouse his mental activity. In his secondary state, the young clergyman enjoyed keenly the antics of the performers, drank beer with pleasure, etc.

After innumerable changes of personality, *generally preceded by sleep*, Hanna merged on June 14 into a curious state resembling mental stupor. To questions put to him and bearing upon his two different personalities he answered very slowly and with great difficulty as though he were in both states at the same time.

[139]

For several days he remained in that condition; gradually his mind became clear and he informed the physicians treating him that he had passed through an intense mental struggle. The two personalities, his normal and his second personalities, arose simultaneously and confronted each other. Each of them was Hanna and yet they were different from each other. He could not choose one only because both were of the same nature; and yet they were too dissimilar to be joined.

Each personality rose and fell in turn. "The struggle," he said to his physicians, "was not so much to choose one as to forget the other. I was trying to find out which I might most easily forget. It seemed impossible to forget one; both tried to persist in consciousness. It seemed as if each memory was stronger than my will, and still I had to determine which to drive away. Just before lunch, yesterday, in the psychological laboratory, I chose the secondary life; it was *strong and fresh* and was able to persist. . . . At that time the question arose whether I could not possibly take both. . . . I decided to accept both lives as mine, a condition that could not be worse than the uncertainty I was in. I then felt that the oft-repeated struggle would ruin my mind. . . . *I am sure both are mine.* They are separate and I cannot yet fit the two

[140]

well together. . . . Secondary and primary states have breaks and intervals in them, as though there were periods of sleep. *The secondary state is stronger and brighter, but not more stable.*"

Harmony gradually re-entered Hanna's mind and the two personalities were merged into a new and healthy one, a compromise between the overworked, overcivilized, over-repressed man of yore and the primitive, uncivilized and unadapted child who for three months had tried to prevail.

In all but one of the cases I have reviewed and in many others which can be found in the literature of the subject, the change in personality was preceded by some "crisis." The crisis is not mentioned in Hanna's case but might have been found if the psychiatrists treating the patient had inquired into the events preceding the "accident." They probably, as was usual in those days (1897), considered the accident as the primary factor in the mental derangement. Hanna's fall may have been, however, what Freud calls a semi-intentional self-inflicted injury.

Ansel Bourne was fleeing from "trouble back there" and "wanted rest," Miss Beauchamp was overcome by "some nervous excitement," Alma Z. was a victim of "overwork," Mary Reynolds had been weakened "by a severe attack."

[141]

In every case the subject, instead of evolving into a more complex, more intelligent, more developed personality, regressed to a more primitive one. The change implied an easier mode of living, fewer duties and responsibilities.

In the case of Alma Z., "The Boy" was obviously trying to save the normal personality from wifely duties. A. Brown, fruit dealer, avoided much of the mental exertion Rev. Bourne had to undergo. Sallie did not have to live up to the intellectual standard Miss Beauchamp had set for herself. Mary Reynolds and Hanna, becoming infants, let the world minister to all their needs.

Every change of personality either took place at night or after a period of sleep, the second personality appearing preferably at night, the normal personality re-appearing preferably in the day time. The second personality assumes the aspect of a protracted dream, and the fact that it appeared at night in so many cases, lends credibility to that view.

The second personality appears in every case as a morbid wish-fulfilment, as a negative striving along a fictitious life-line, along the line of least resistance. Every one of the subjects observed was probably a person harassed and worn out by either monotonous tasks or an exaggerated sense of duty.

[142]

The playful or infantile personalities into which they merged temporarily, took abnormally the vacation they themselves should have taken normally.

They all had repressed, if not over-repressed, the old Adam, and the old Adam avenged himself by bursting forth and assuming the upper hand. How many cases of so-called "insanity" are simply due to the persistency of a second personality which happens to be too violent or absurd to be tolerable in its environment. A patient now confined at Ward's Island became insane after being hit on the head by a small tin can which did not even abrase the skin. A journeyman before the accident, he has become a famous opera singer and holds frequent conversations with God. He, too, has entered an easier life, doing no manual labour, enjoying a prestige he could never aspire to in his former occupation and unburdened of the care of his family; the fulfilment of a dream which may have originated in the unconscious moments following the accident; another case in which the accident seems to have been a "pretext" seized by the unconscious rather than a positive cause.

The more things we lack in our waking states, the more things we shall expect and receive from our dreams, but many of our dream accomplishments are archaic, regressive, infantile. Not infrequently when our conscious self deprives itself of gratifications which human nature craves, our unconscious self overpowers it and proceeds to lead even in our waking states a more human, more comfortable, sort of life. Like all the results of violent upheavals, however, that life is likely to be unbalanced and unadapted to our environment. The ascetic saints who, in their scorn of the flesh, fled into the desert, were a prey to horrible halluci- nations in which they beheld all the obscenities which consciously they had been avoiding but for which they unconsciously had been craving.

Our archaic, unconscious self is a lusty caveman whose cravings modern civilization can no longer satisfy. He must, however, be appeased now and then by being given a sop of some sort. Starving him can only bring about his revolt; his attempts to free himself may mean sick headaches, hysteria, obsessions, phobias, "insanity" or the appearance of a new man in the body of the old, the domination of a second personality for a more or less extended period of time.

BIBLIOGRAPHY

Sidis and Goodhart, "Multiple Personality" (Apple- ton) will supply the reader with a history of the best known cases. Neither of the authors is a psychoanalyst, one of them, Dr. Sidis, being in fact, bitterly opposed to that science.

Their observations, however, are very valuable and do not in any way contradict those made by exponents of psychoanalysis.

CHAPTER V. HOW ONE WOMAN BECAME INSANE

Psychoanalysts seldom have the opportunity of treating any of the "great psychoses." The patient who has lost all insight into his mental condition is generally confined in an institution and few insane asylums have analysts on their medical staff.

One case treated by Dr. Kempf at St. Elizabeth Hospital, Washington, D. C., offers good evidence that many apparently "desperate" cases could be cured by the psychoanalytic technique.

If an abstract of that case is presented to the reader, it is not merely owing to the success which crowned Dr. Kempf's efforts, but because it offers, besides, a striking and grewsome picture of the process by which people are at times "driven to insanity."

It shows how well-meaning associates, lacking in sympathy and understanding, beset with many prejudices and affected by complexes of their own, may gradually make reality so unbearable for a weaker individual that he unconsciously seeks to

[146]

escape it by the door which leads to an insane asylum.

The various relapses which Kempf's patient suffered before she regained her normal balance illustrate perhaps more impressively than any other detail of the case that process of abnormal escape from unpleasant situations.

The influence which education may have in determining the content of psychopathic fancies was made very clear by the analysis of Kempf's patient.

The patient was a young woman of twenty-four, married and the mother of a child. She was the youngest of several children.

Her father was an engineer, a hard-worker, saving to the point of being stingy and obsessed by the fear of being destitute in his old age. He loved his children but tended to conflict with them owing to his prudishness. All sexual topics were taboo in his home. He berated his daughters when they sat with their legs crossed, he objected to their wearing kimonos. He owned some houses in a distant city which were for a time, through no fault of his own, converted into brothels.

In his later years he depended upon his oldest daughter to manage his affairs and persistently inclined to treat the youngest as a child. At the

[147]

time of the patient's illness, he was about seventy years old and suffering from chronic gastritis.

The mother was a "nervous," kind, home loving woman, tall and heavy, and extremely fond of eating. She, like her husband, encouraged her oldest daughter to be self-reliant and, on the other hand, trained her youngest daughter to depend upon her in every way, introducing her to visitors as the baby. She never allowed the "baby" to have any initiative and imposed her will upon her in all matters, telling her what style and material to select for her clothes, what to wear for the day, how to act, to whom to talk, etc.

Like her husband, she also excluded from her conversation all matters pertaining to sex and never tolerated any intimate confidence on the part of her children. The patient was whipped at the age of eleven for asking her mother about the meaning of a word she read in a toilet and for relating to her her fancies in connection with that word.

The patient's oldest sister was mentally and physically very like the mother and she, too, demanded constant submission to her decisions and opinions on the part of the patient.

In other words the patient's training had unfitted her for self-reliance and efficiency in real life. She was perfectly satisfied with that arrangement and even was inclined to treat her own inefficiency and irresponsibility as a joke. She was a lazy and rather obese type of girl. Her education was never planned systematically and she missed many school days on whimsical pretexts.

Her early curiosity in regard to sexual problems only met with rebuke and on several occasions with punishment.

Her parents' prudishness only increased her interest in all things pertaining to reproduction. She watched excitedly cats, dogs, chickens, horses and derived much secret enjoyment from her observation of their sexual behaviour. On the other hand she would be morbidly embarrassed by the sight of a woman nursing a child.

Her father considered it indecent for her to sit on his lap. When her sister began to menstruate and she tried to secure information as to that phenomenon, her mother scolded her and sent her to her room. She felt then that she lived on a plane beneath her mother and her sister and she developed a distinct feeling of inferiority.

She trained herself never to ask questions because they might expose her thoughts and she would have remained in absolute ignorance of sexual facts but for the romantic stories told her by a coloured maid who had been employed once in a house of prostitution. Those stories simply set her imagination on fire and far from enlightening her, caused her to derive sexual suggestions from almost everything in her environment, the behaviour of her father and mother, the sight of attractive women, etc.

At twenty-one, she married a young man whose family was in almost every respect quite the opposite of her own.

His father was also an engineer, but younger than the patient's father, a free spender and fond of gay parties.

The patient's mother-in-law was a handsome woman with a girlish figure, small feet and ankles, well dressed, who had travelled a good deal and had a wide range of interests. She was proud of her youthful appearance and dieted in order to keep herself attractive looking.

The patient's husband was a slender man who at thirty had the figure of a wiry, active boy of twenty. He also was an engineer, ambitious, earnest, spoiled by his mother, and at times irritable and impulsive.

During their engagement, the patient never allowed her fiancé to kiss her or to put his arm around her. She was terribly upset and almost gave him up when he confessed to her that he had

[150]

had a hard struggle with his desire to masturbate and had consorted with other girls. She never communicated her wish to desert him to any one then but later in her psychose felt sure that their marriage was not legal.

At that time she finally demanded that her mother enlighten her as to the origin of children and she felt extremely shocked by her mother's explanation and always hated her in later life for having deceived her so long.

After the novelty of their relation and the excitement attendant upon the first months of married life had worn away, her husband began to be disturbed by what he called "asinine thoughts." He could not understand why dainty feet, hairless limbs, small firm breasts and a small abdomen (his mother's characteristics) should prove so attractive to him and why large soft breasts, a large abdomen, heavy feet and ankles and hairy limbs (his wife's characteristics) should prove sexually depressing.

He was undoubtedly conscious of his mother-fixation and in his more or less conscious endeavour to escape incest had selected for his mate the opposite type of a woman. His mother-fixation was clearly revealed by incestuous dreams which pursued him even after his marriage.

He was greatly relieved later when told of the simple biological significance of such dreams. Realizing obscurely to what causes his growing sexual indifference to his wife was due, he tried to induce her to diet, to exercise (in order to reduce her abdomen and breasts) and to remove the hair from her ankles. After a while she gave up those practices which would have made her a little more similar to the mother-image and became careless about her appearance.

The two families did not harmonize at all. Her family appeared too coarse and bigoted to her husband's family which in turn was scorned by her family for its freer views and extravagance. The two families naturally made the unfortunate young woman their common battle ground because she was weak and unsophisticated.

Her husband caused her much distress by threatening to leave her if she lost her beauty, if she did not take better care of her appearance, or did not write to him daily when he was away.

Her sexual life was naturally very unsatisfactory and she masturbated during her pregnancy, after which she was overwhelmed with shame. To make matters worse, her sister told her that masturbation was a symptom of insanity. She was obsessed by the fear that her child might inherit her bad habits. When the child was born and her husband showed a good deal of indifference to it, his threats to leave her caused her more and more anxiety.

Both families resumed their strife over the child. Her mother-in-law insisted upon plenty of fresh air for the infant and her own mother protested that they were freezing it. The patient's mother finally assumed complete charge of the child and treated it like her own.

When her husband was away, his mother berated her for not travelling with him; her mother objected to this because she would neglect the baby by going to meet her husband out of town.

She was made to regard herself as a failure, both as a wife and as a mother. Her husband, thoroughly frightened but well-meaning, decided then to educate her. For that purpose he gave her an absurd book on "sexology" filled with moralizing platitudes on masturbation and perversions. The only conclusion she drew from reading that drivel was that she was a pervert and a degenerate, absolutely unfit to raise her child, and that her child was doomed to become abnormal.

She had fits of crying and depression and often told her family she wished she, her husband and baby were dead. She spoke of her husband remarrying and asked her sister to take care of the baby when she married her husband. She indulged more and more in masturbation and began to speak of it openly. Delusions appeared. She thought people sneered at her "as if she was passing disgusting odours." She insisted that she was not her father's daughter but a prostitute in a house kept by her father; she thought she saw a picture of herself in tights in the *Police Gazette*; she was afraid medicines might contain poison. Finally she drank tincture of iodine in an attempt to kill herself and thereupon was taken to a sanatorium.

In that institution which she, in her delusions, considered as a house of prostitution, some stupid nurses yielded to the temptation of playing upon her sexual fears and told her many weird sadistic stories of immorality. Pursued by erotic fancies she tried hard to resist her cravings and adopted no end of devices to save herself from masturbation. She experienced a profound sense of her sinfulness and her letters to her husband contained many references to her worthlessness, to the fact that she had ruined her baby, etc.

She was then removed from the sanatorium to St. Elizabeth Hospital.

Her husband was deeply affected by his wife's mental derangement and was conscious of his responsibility for her depression and anxiety. His first visits were very cautiously conducted and he always sought advice as to what to say to her. She reacted in a gratifying way to his kind attitude.

She gradually accorded Dr. Kempf her confidence and learned to depend upon him for assurance and encouragement. She became adjusted to a higher level of interest.

Suddenly, however, she began to regress, reverting to her prostitution fancies. The cause was not far to seek.

One day her husband, losing his patience, had in the course of a visit threatened again to leave her if she did not get well. She learnt also that he had been drinking.

Some time afterward she had another regression which was traced again to some stupid statements made by her husband. Her mother had died and willed all her property to the patient's father which necessitated the signature of all the heirs, including the patient. Her husband had carried the will in his pocket for several days trying to decide whether or not he would sign it. He brought up the whole family conflict again and told the patient that her mother must have been *insane* when she made that will. They were together at the patient's dance when it occurred and she changed in a few minutes

[155]

from a state of hopefulness and promise to one of serious confusion and inaccessibility.

This lasted nearly two weeks and then she became more cheerful.

Then the family difficulties were once more depressed upon her by her husband, sister and father and this time she regressed almost completely to a prenatal attitude. She was afraid of being smothered in boxes, of being passed into the toilet with feces, she had all sorts of terrifying hallucinations.

Her dreams, however, showed affective trends which suggested that a reconstruction was possible. She developed more and more interest in her environment, her child, her husband. She gathered much insight into her condition and could analyse her delusions very skilfully.

About the twenty-third week she had rallied so far that a nurse took her out to visit her people. Then the old family quarrel about spending money flared up again. The patient wished to change the arrangement of the furniture and her sister, as domineering as ever, prevented her from asserting herself even during her brief stay at home. She returned to the hospital angry and worried.

She had too much insight by that time, owing to the psychoanalytic treatment she had been undergoing, to regress very far. She recovered and was finally discharged.

Two months afterward, a crisis confronted her again. She was pregnant and some members of her family were urging her to resort to an abortion. She managed to assert herself, however, and bore the child.

When she was discharged from the hospital, she seemed to be uncomfortable about two things, her inability to find a religion which was free from dogma and hypocrisy and a feeling that her education was not ample. Kempf gave her a rather indefinite reply on the subject of religion but accorded more serious consideration to her feelings of inferiority about her education.

Her education had been badly supervised and her conception of her fitness as a woman was not commensurate with the magnificent affections of a practical nature which were natural to her. She had become more of a woman in her sympathies and insight than the average social light. She had a keen insight into the affective mechanism of people surrounding her.

In order to free herself from her feeling of inferiority she read, upon Kempf's advice, biographies of famous women and gradually came to the conclusion that much of her suffering had been due to her repression of her affections. She determined to join the movement for woman's emancipation.

Her husband had to be educated too. Attentive and kind to her, he was still too completely enthralled by his mother-fixation to co-operate with Kempf very faithfully. He could not restrain his tendency to criticize his wife and to show displeasure over her diet, her careless way of dressing, etc. Kempf told him explicitly that he should not suppress, among other things, her interest in feminism, but frankly support it. He agreed to do so but was not quite able to keep his word.

The patient, however, in spite of all the pressure which both families tried again to bring to bear upon her, asserted herself.

She met their arguments with the statements that she must use her own judgment "because her physician had insisted upon it," and that she did not care what they had to say. She could not please everybody and no matter what happened she knew her physician respected her personal integrity and sincerity.

The way in which she managed her second pregnancy and the rearrangement of her household were very encouraging. The only distressing note was a statement she made that if any hopeless family estrangement should arise she would kill herself.

Therein lurked the possibility of a fateful regression to the lowest possible level, the fatal level, for the committing of suicide is a regression to the eternal mother, an effort to return to the ancient state of intrauterine peace, comfort and dependence.

Now, four years after her discharge from the hospital, she is in excellent mental condition, working out most of her plans to her heart's desire and taking good care of her two children.

Intelligent, sympathetic re-education, reducing her feeling of inferiority; the reliance she could place in a well known psychiatrist understanding her better than any member of her family and whose opinions had naturally more weight than that of any one else in her environment have enabled her to become herself at last.

A perusal of this remarkable case furnishes the reader with concrete applications of various statements contained in the chapters on the Love Life and the Sexual Enlightenment of Children.

The puritanical father and mother who in their fear of facts allowed their daughters to remain in ignorance of the sexual truth until a former inmate of a house of prostitution brought them the most spurious and romantic form of enlightenment are familiar figures. The baneful influence of a prudish father continually throwing obscene suggestions into the minds of his children by his very efforts to instil "modesty" into them is graphically illustrated.

This case also offers us a demonstration of the effects which a man's mother-fixation can have upon that man's sexual partner, causing her to experience a sense of physical inferiority because to his complex-beset mind, the mother type only can represent feminine attraction and arouse his desire.

The striking change which the crisis brought about in the patient's personality and in her attitude to life, makes good food for thought. It is difficult to avoid the conclusions that AFTER BEING INSANE and recovering she was better fitted for life, and had become a more interesting human type than before the onset of her neurosis.

To one who realizes that recovery from a severe neurosis means the acquisition of an enormous amount of insight into, not only one's own thinking functions and motives, but into the psychology of one's associates as well, it will be evident that many persons who lived through such a terrible experience may have developed a more robust mentality than they ever had.

Unfortunately that view is not held by many people and the individual who was unfortunate enough to require treatment in an institution for the insane comes back to his former environment bearing an undefinable stigma. People are afraid of him and expect him to "go crazy" again at some time or other. And their fears are, if not justified, at least often realized. The insane man who made a recovery sometimes becomes insane again because he has been discouraged in his fight for reality by the very same people who once drove him into insanity.

Kempf's patient having it dinned constantly in her ears by two absolutely dissimilar groups of people that she was crazy finally followed the line of least resistance and yielded to their absurd pronouncement. The pressure of such environmental forces together with the fact that the patient was actually insane once and may have a few lingering doubts about his complete recovery, may succeed in sending him back to the institution from which he was discharged.

As Kempf writes, "The thoughtless attitude of the people is to be changed by educating them to have as much confidence in those who have recovered from mental diseases as they have in those who recover from other diseases, in order to help the patient to be less fearful of being distrusted

[161]

and disrespected. Both sides of this procedure have essentially a therapeutic value in that they are conducive to an easier and more durable recovery for the patient as well as exerting a humanizing influence on the people. Hence the procedure should be an important part of the therapeutic method, a permanent, outstanding feature of the hospital life of the patient and the means of maintaining social contact between the hospital and the community."

Finally the method employed by Kempf in restoring his patient to a normal condition exposes the absurdity of herding the insane by the thousands in institutions where nature is mainly relied upon to bring about a cure. Let the average man, Kempf writes, imagine what distress he would suffer and what changes of character he would undergo if he were confined indefinitely in a hospital ward, his judgment discredited, and forced to associate constantly with twenty to fifty other worrying, unhappy people, many of whom had lost control of themselves and become sexually perverse either overtly or in fancy. The universal answer would be that the experience would soon become unendurable to the sane man or woman and cause nothing less than prolonged misery and suffering.

[162]

The hospital for mental diseases, he concludes, should be a first class vocational university for the practical re-education and rehabilitation of the people who have become abnormal and unable to adapt themselves to their social obligations' and the social laws, due to their incompatible cravings and previous unsuitable education and training.

Such a plan would require for its realization a considerable increase in the number of physicians, nurses, attendants, and vocational and athletic trainers. This would at first appear very expensive, but, as Kempf remarks, owing to the great reduction in the duration of the average patient's illness, and the increase in recoveries, the annual cost would be greatly reduced after a few years.

Eighty per cent. of the mentally diseased, he thinks, could be cured if properly treated. This applies, of course, to cases in which there is no destruction of nervous tissues.

Furthermore, the asylum would lose its depressing, ominous stigma and many patients in the incipient stage would be influenced to come and seek treatment before their condition had become chronic or incurable. What with the many who would not become insane owing to preventive measures, and the many insane who could be helped to regain their mental balance, the population of insane asylums would be greatly reduced by adopting Kempf's suggestions.

BIBLIOGRAPHY

A complete report of this interesting case will be found in the *Psychoanalytic Review* for January, 1919, under the title "The Psychoanalytic Treatment of Dementia Praecox" by Dr. Edward J. Kempf.

Dr. Kempf's theories are discussed in the last chapter of the present book. His ideas on the management of hospitals for the insane, which are very progressive, have been published under the title "Important Needs of Hospitals for Mental Disease," *New York Medical Journal,* July 5, 1919.

CHAPTER VI. THE NEUROTIC ASPECTS OF WAR

Civilization eliminates many of nature's wasteful methods and reduces to a minimum the friction between human beings. It modifies individual habits and transforms them into clan or herd habits, later into national habits. It teaches individuals a certain measure of solidarity.

The herd bands together to repel aggressors of a different species; wolves hunt in packs and do not attack one another; flocks of migrating birds wait till a tired member of the flock is ready to resume the voyage. The advantages of solidarity, however, are only obscurely realized by the majority of animals and when no emergency compels them to realize them, we see them often murdering one another to secure one favourite female or a larger allotment of the available food.

Man, likewise, seldom adapts himself permanently to standards which are very superior socially to the purely individual standard. His ego, sex and safety urges can be repressed for a certain length of time, mainly out of necessity, physical or social, but they are constantly striving for direct or indirect expression, sometimes through chance actions, cruel or obscene wit, day and night dreams.

Not only does civilized community life compel a repression of the urges which is contrary to primitive human nature, but the demands it makes are growing by leaps and bounds. Such demands are growing faster than men, the world over, can make their urge repression really efficient.

Thus a constantly increasing emotional strain is created which manifests itself in abnormal ways among the weaker members of the community. The robust and well-fed generally manage to remain normal regardless of the physical and mental risks they run. The inferior organisms either break down under the strain or defy the customs of the community and pay the penalty or they seek the line of least resistance and submit in appearance.

The population of the world, for that reason, consists of many more simulators than truly adapted human beings. Restrictions are burdensome to them but they either conceal the fact as a matter of policy or in many cases are ashamed of their own impatience and do not even confess it to themselves.

In sudden crises, however, all the pent-up urges

are likely to break through with a violence which astonishes us.

In times of war, we cannot help expressing our surprise at the amount of savagery and cruelty displayed by the victorious armies, but that surprise simply shows our ignorance of the actual state of things. It is not, as Freud suggests, that people sink very low in war times; they never were as high in peace times as we imagined them to be.

We all spend one-half of our life regressing to the archaic, individual, uncivilized level; for as soon as we fall asleep, we discard our morality, our ethics, and all our repressions even as we cast off our clothes, and indulge in a riot of egotistical and sexual gratification through our dreams.

The only thing which generally holds us back in our waking time is, either the fear of punishment, direct or indirect, the fear of jail or of social ostracism, or a clear realization of the financial and social advantages vouchsafed by apparent conformism.

As soon as war is declared, the terrible tension is released and most of our animal instincts find gratification; that gratification entails no loss of caste, prestige or money; on the contrary. In war, the whole community regresses to the animal

[167]

level and punishes the individual who refuses to regress with the herd.

Every animal is born with a craving for food, which very soon evolves into a craving for power, power being the shortest road to more plentiful and better food secured with the least possible amount of exertion.

Civilized man no longer starts out with a club to dispute dangerous beasts of prey or other hunters of a different clan their right to hunt, nor does he send out his slaves to run down game. He has covered the brutality of the quest under civilized veneer and manages to give partial satisfaction to his archaic instincts in ways which do not inflict too much suffering upon his environment.

War removes the inhibitions introduced by modern business methods. Every nation wishes to conquer some piece of land for reasons which, at times, can well masquerade as humanitarian ones, as for instance the necessity of freeing some "enslaved" race which we hope to dominate, or in order to "open up" markets, or to free men of our race who, in a more or less dim past, were submitted to forceful annexation by another race, etc.

Whatever the pretence, the result is the same: all the individuals of one community are exhilar-

[168]

ated by the prospect of starting out to plunder the neighbour's land.

As a matter of fact, very few members of the herd, not one out of ten thousand, will be benefited in any way by the foray, and those few, bankers and traders, never take part in the expedition, but the masses of the fighters enjoy the fact that they are engaged in an adventurous undertaking of a primitive, archaic type, which in ordinary times would be highly unethical but which now is authorized, financed and idealized by the community.

The civilized nation has regressed to the level of the robber herd of the caveman period. We may point out that in legends and in the real life of backward communities, the successful robber is a romantic, privileged character, to whom the usual standards do not apply.

At such times, some members of the community regress even lower than the herd level.

The herd on the war path is hunting for the herd. No single member of the herd will profit by the conquests achieved, and the sense of herd solidarity is not abolished. The profiteer, on the other hand, is entirely devoid of that sense. While the herd is hunting, he does not hesitate to starve it if he can only corner the herd's food supply and then sell it at the price his power can dictate and thus gratify his appetite.

Profiteering is individualism gone mad. Like the herd's craving for blood and spoils, it may assume a righteous mask: supplies are difficult to secure "on account of the war," those who protest are branded as unpatriotic for they lack the "spirit of self-sacrifice," etc.

Lying and deceit, two neurotic devices of the negative life, and universally tabooed in the individual's life, become praiseworthy in war times and especially indulged in by the men who prepare wars, the diplomats. Diplomacy's greatest accomplishment consists in attaining an object without letting any outsider suspect it and preferably convincing outsiders that an entirely different object is being sought.

The greatest diplomats were those who not only had the greatest capacity for deceiving the rulers at whose court they were accredited but for covering up their traces so carefully that they actually gained their confidence.

In war times, lying about the enemy is not unethical. It is, on the contrary, highly commendable as it sustains the morale of fighters and civilians alike.

Exhibitionism is another deeply ingrained and

[170]

infantile craving of all races, made up in equal doses of sex and ego. The males of many species parade around the females at mating time, trying to arouse their sexuality and at the same time probably frightening away other males.

War offers many excellent excuses for a display of exhibitionism.

The warrior is clothed in a uniform which once presented a dazzling array of colours and in certain cases was enhanced by precious metals, and which, drab as it has become today, for reasons of safety, is sufficient to place those wearing it on a higher plane than the civilian.

The wearing of a uniform places all soldiers in one category in which every individual is supposed to be healthy and vigorous and hence fit for purposes of reproduction.

The females respond properly and we see thousands of service clubs in which young women, some of them imitating the males and wearing uniforms, foster the men's belief that they are privileged characters; some of the women belonging to "society" converse or dance with men whom they would absolutely ignore if they cast off the distinguishing regalia of the fighting male and donned civilian's clothes.

In war times, the desire for promiscuous intercourse which lurks in every human being can be indulged in without calling forth undue criticism. The most jealous husbands are compelled to approve of their wives' "war activities."

The war regression is a boon to all the weak members of the community who are anxious to regress to a childlike level but are compelled by economic necessity to remain on the adult level. The useless, the shiftless, who for lack of intelligence or perseverance, never were able to accomplish anything positive, who have been a butt for much scorn and contumely, are suddenly enabled to play a striking part in their little world by enlisting or being drafted.

Not only are their failures forgotten, but an escape from stern reality is vouchsafed them. All of life's responsibilities are now shifted to the state. The state feeds, clothes and shelters them and assumes the charge of their dependents. Nothing that befalls the enlisted man's family can affect him very deeply, for as soon as he joins the colours his responsibility ceases.

As soon as he dons a uniform, the useless and shiftless weakling becomes an object of attention on the part of women, even as the worthier males. That the sexual element plays a greater part in the devotion women show to fighters than a spirit of

[172]

self-sacrifice is well proved by the fact that while social clubs had more volunteers at their disposal than they could possibly employ, the hospitals of New York City during the epidemic of influenza of 1919 were unable to find nurses. Although by that time the war emergency was over one nurse in ward B1 at Bellevue Hospital had to take care of as many as fifty patients for 12 hours at a time.

One of the features constantly reported in war news are stories of sexual license and violence.

The sex instinct, submitted to a terrible repression in peace times, breaks through when so many other inhibitions are removed. In all epochs of history the fighting man's morality has been the subject of special allowances. In the past, one of war's sequels was the seizing of the defeated enemy's women by the victorious tribe. Moses told his men to keep for themselves all the virgins of the Midianite tribe which they had defeated. The enemy's wife or sister has never been sacred. Training camps and garrison towns have always been known as centres of promiscuous sexual intercourse.

Another one of the infantile activities which is carefully regulated from an early age and whose haphazard gratification is severely repressed is the anal and vesical activity, the passing of feces and

[173]

urine. A regression to such activities in their infantile form is reported quite frequently in war times. The invading soldiers often defile in the most nauseating way the quarters which they occupy, not respecting even at times religious vessels or other paraphernalia of the enemy's cult.

The necessities of the national defence enable any one with a neurotic strain of cruelty to satisfy his craving even in his immediate environment, without regard for the law of the herd.

Thousands of people spy on one another, listen to conversations in public places and, whenever hearing something suspicious, have the offender arraigned, if not dragged in a spectacular way to the police station.

This is a manifestation of the egotistical negativism which, unable to achieve anything, lowers other people's level through disparagement and destructive hostility.

War allows us to insult any one we dislike by calling him a traitor or a seditious person and denouncing him to the police authorities. If he is higher than we are, we "get even" with him, if he is our equal we make him our inferior, if he belongs to a lower social rank, we can then express our scorn without appearing snobbish.

Atrocities are being committed in every war by

[174]

the victorious armies. Whether they assume the form of cruel treatment of civilians or consist in using trench gas, liquid flame or other means of torture, makes very little difference. Every one pretends to experience a profound indignation on reading about them, but no one ever suggests anything but reprisals, retaliation.

In peace times, we do not disembowel Jack the Ripper because he resorted to that frightful form of violence, we do not burn alive the man who set fire to a house. In war the path of regression to primitive cruelty is wide open "for the sake of example."

Primitive savages wno wish something, represent it dramatically, sprinkling the ground to bring rain from the clouds, burning some one in effigy, etc.

In war times, the population is made to behold at every step lurid posters representing the annihilation of the foe. Rabid statements are made vociferously as to what we shall do to the enemy, how completely we are going to crush him, to hit him so hard that he shall never rise again. In other words the task which confronts the nation is constantly represented as being successfully performed and brought to a glorious ending.

There is also in the rage with which the community destroys the things symbolical of the enemy a

[175]

regression to the period of infamy which Ferenczi calls the period of belief in the omnipotence of thought and magic gestures.

By forbidding the display of certain flags, by placing a ban on books and publications printed in the enemy's language, by interfering with musical performances in which an enemy performer is taking part or at which the works of an enemy would be given, certain neurotics think they can destroy the enemy more completely.

Whatever symbolizes the enemy and makes him present symbolically is done away with. Here we behold a process akin to the withdrawal from reality in dementia praecox and to the ostrich's habit of burying his head in the sand.

Such prohibitions show a regression to the belief in magic, a decided evasion of reality and a flight along the line of least resistance.

Intolerance is the most marked characteristic phenomenon of war times. It also characterizes severe cases of neurosis.

One cannot discuss with a neurotic. The psychiatrist who tries to bring insight into his patient's mind would lose the battle at once if he began by telling him that his story is absurd.

The thing to do is to let the neurotic tell his

[176]

story in his own way, to throw light gradually on the spurious evidence on which he has built it and thus to disintegrate it. But the more absurd the obsession, the harder the neurotic will fight to have his version accepted. The hopelessly insane who knows he is a king or god easily resorts to violence when some one betrays scepticism.

The neurotic may obscurely feel that his story is wrong and cannot be defended. Hence his impotence is easily enraged and he avoids all discussions in which he could not hold his own.

In war times, rabid neurotics who monopolize the title of patriot do not allow any one to discuss the war or any of its problems. If they were sure of their ground they would gladly confute doubters, but being thrall to their emotions they have to follow the line of least resistance. "Only traitors," they say quite finally, "discuss the merits of a war after war has been started."

Intolerance is the last refuge of the loser. Having no strong argument wherewith to silence you, he hits you on the mouth.

The consequences of the wholesale regression which takes place during war are interesting to examine.

The states engaged in war disregard all the eth-

[177]

ical rules which have established themselves as the fundamentals of behaviour in all civilized communities.

They lie, they practise deceit at home and abroad, they deprive people of their freedom of speech, they sentence dissenters to incredibly long jail terms, etc.

The masses of the population can only reach one conclusion: that is that, while ethics, morality and honesty are very fine in theory, they are non-existent when tried by the reality test.

Ethics, morality and honesty are valuable when no emergency has to be coped with. As soon as the great emergency of war arises, however, the state sets them aside as useless or detrimental.

Hence ethics, morality and honesty seem to have only a relative value, not an absolute one and the danger is that, when the masses instilled with that doctrine of relativity want something very badly, they may also act as the state acts in emergencies.

An enormous amount of savagery lingers in people's attitudes following a war. Men of a conservative type who, before a war, would boast of their human feelings and deprecate all forms of violence, are heard suggesting violence against their opponents. "Shoot them at sunrise," "Get the rope," "Shoot them first and try them next," are

[178]

the favourite expressions of neurotics brutalized by the war spirit.

Their opponents, their enemies are transformed through mental juggling into enemies of the country, and hence deserving death. This is a typically infantile attitude. The child powerless against a stronger boy throws in his face a desperate "I wish you'd die." Here is again the line of least resistance. Nothing will save us from our opponent except his death. We then make that death a public necessity.

The politician who goes about the country preaching a summary execution for those who disagree with him, is unknowingly proclaiming their absolute superiority and his absolute incapacity to fight them fairly in a civilized way.

The constant charge of intended violence brought by certain men against groups they intend to persecute is, generally speaking, a projection of their own murderous cravings upon their intended victims. Suspecting a man of violence is the simplest excuse for submitting him to violence. By pretending that we saw a man put his hand to his hip pocket we can always plead self-defence when we do him to death.

The description of many raids made upon the locals of labour organizations in recent months reveals that the leaders of those raids were not bent so much on preventing or punishing violence as on indulging without danger to themselves in an orgy of violence.

Raiders entering premises ostensibly to seek damaging evidence have been known to smash everything in the rooms from electric lamps to mechanical pianos and typewriting machines.

It will be noticed also that all great wars are followed by epidemics. They are generally attributed to unsanitary conditions induced by the destruction of hygienic appliances, the presence of dead bodies, the weakening of the population by famine, etc.

The importance of all these factors could not be denied by any rational scientist. Another factor, however, should be added to the list. When almost all the forms of approved regression made available by the war emergency have been removed, when active negativism has become impossible, passive negativism enters into play. The neurotic who could satisfy his ego through exhibitionism and sadism and become by the performance of some simple standardized actions a centre of interest has to find some other means of dominating neurotically his environment.

This is easily done by assuming unconsciously,

[180]

(not by any means consciously) the symptoms of a simple, seasonable disease, whose description is to be found in all the papers, and in that way regress to a helpless level, into a privileged class which enjoys every one's sympathy and help, receives medical care, is talked about, is never touched by suspicion of malingering, owing to the prevalence of the disturbance and is, for the time being, removed from and protected against reality into which it may fall back gradually.

BIBLIOGRAPHY

FREUD, S.—"Reflections on War and Death" (Moffat, Yard) and WHITE, W. A.—"Thoughts of a Psychiatrist on the War and After" (Hoeber) are two small and most readable books which show one Austrian and one American psychiatrist reaching practically the same conclusions from their observations of the world war.

IV. SLEEP AND DREAMS

CHAPTER I: SLEEP, SLEEPLESSNESS AND NIGHTMARES

The most common explanation for the fact that we go to sleep is that we are tired and need rest.

A close examination of the organism in its sleeping condition fails to lend plausibility to that theory.

The heart continues to beat and to send the blood stream on its course through the body. The lungs continue to gather in oxygen, the liver to accumulate glycogen. The stomach and bowels keep on digesting and eliminating, our beard keeps on growing, all our glands keep on producing various secretions. Some, like our sweat glands, are infinitely more active in our sleep than in our waking state. Our mind does not rest by any means for we probably dream every minute of every night.

Our vagotonic activities, that is, the autonomic nervous activities which upbuild the body and tend to perpetuate the race, are infinitely stronger in sleep than the sympathicotonic activities which restrain them.

Our sense organs are as acutely sensitive in sleep

as in the waking state, for the slightest stimulus brings about a reaction of some sort, mostly in the form of a dream.

Besides the fact that we do not move our arms and legs, or at least move them very little while asleep, it is rather difficult to mention any part of the body which actually "rests" in sleep.

The explanation that sleep enables us to eliminate from the organism the various fatigue products is not convincing, for inactivity not accompanied by unconsciousness would enable the blood to carry off those products as completely as inactivity does when accompanied by unconsciousness.

The same answer could be given to those who claim that in sleep we store up again the substances (for instance sugar) which waking activity has spent lavishly.

It is not clear why unconsciousness would help that process.

What is it, then, which a conscious state does not give us and which we only find in unconsciousness?

Only by studying dreams will we find a satisfactory answer to that question.

Dreams secure gratification for thousands of expressed or repressed desires; dreams find solutions, some of them absurd, some of them acceptable, to problems which have puzzled us in our waking hours; dreams, even though they SEEM frightening, painful or humiliating, always fulfil some conscious or unconscious wish. The process is very obvious in gross sexual dreams, less obvious in dreams which cloak themselves with complicated symbolism, and not at all obvious in nightmares.

When dreams transform the dreamer into an irresistible Don Juan or a millionaire, he is quite willing to accept the theory of wish fulfilment. When a young girl dreams that she is pursued or bitten by a dog she may feel rather sceptical as to the universal application of that theory.

Most of our dreams, however, are symbolical, that is, they say what they have to say in a language which we ourselves do not understand, paradoxical as it may seem.

We throw shoes and rice at newlyweds without actually understanding the meaning of that act. Yet we are expressing in that symbolical way a wish which is quite appropriate to the occasion, and which we would not dare to express in any other way.

Shoes are a symbol of the female genitals, rice the symbol of the male fecundating element. Shoes and rice have that meaning not only in more

[187]

or less fantastic and in accurate dream books but in all the folklore of all races (rice being in certain cases replaced by wheat or other local cereal).

Thus we express symbolically the wish that the newly married pair may be prolific, a wish which the delicacy or hypocrisy of our modern civilization would not enable us to formulate too directly.

And curiously enough the symbol which unconsciously we understand quite well, has been invested by many with a different conscious meaning. Many people whom I asked for their interpretation of that custom answered, "Well, I suppose it is meant to say: 'May the young couple always have enough to eat and shoes to wear.'"

The orange blossoms which crown brides were originally an allusion to the great fertility of the orange tree which bears fruit twice a year. The shyness which the modern mind shows in the presence of "brutal" sexual facts has gradually placed the stress on the colour of those blossoms and has caused them to symbolize maidenly purity, which after all is only another sexual fact.

In both cases, the repression of sexual instincts by the growing complexity of community life has managed to add a conscious meaning to a ritual which has an entirely different unconscious meaning.

[188]

But it is the unconscious meaning which symbols retain in our dream life, for then the repression is infinitely less powerful.

Dreams aim at giving us absolute freedom of action and expression but they do not always succeed completely in spite of the symbolical mask which they assume in so many cases.

Life's repressions may be so severe that even in sleep the pent-up urges encounter obstacles to their gratification. The result is anxiety dreams, popularly known as nightmares, which are at times the source of a great deal of suffering, until the subject understands their symbolic meaning.

The woman pursued in her dreams by snakes, or trampled upon by horses, or bitten by dogs, etc., is one suffering from lack of sexual gratification and attaining that satisfaction in her sleep in symbolical ways. A subject obsessed by suicidal ideas but who did not wish to leave his family unprovided for, owing to the suicide clause in his insurance policy, would dream night after night that he was put to death for some crime, thus accomplishing his object without causing his dependents any financial loss.

While dreams of being trampled down by animals or being put to death are not to be considered at first glance as constituting the fulfilment of

[189]

wishes, the first anxiety dream is clearly a symbolic form of wish fulfilment, the second, when interpreted with the help of the subject, appears a simple solution of a problem which at one time agitated the subject's mind and hence is also a wish fulfilment.

The function of sleep, then, is to compensate us for all the things we must forego in our waking life, for all the desires we must repress in order to conform to civilized standards. Sleep is a means of escape from reality and from the monotony of existence.

The more complex civilization becomes the more necessary sleep becomes and the more frequent are mental disturbances due to lack of sleep. At the same time, it must be noticed that certain people whose lives are extremely strenuous do not require as much sleep as others do who lead a much more peaceful existence. Napoleon hardly ever slept more than four hours before he reached the Island of Saint Helena. He then slept much longer. Edison does not require more sleep than Napoleon. Many other famous men managed to live a healthy life while taking very little rest.

But those men also led a life in which they fulfilled almost all their wishes. Their work was not drudgery. Napoleon's life was a continuous

[190]

romance of the most exciting sort. Edison's inventive genius vouchsafes his ego innumerable forms of satisfaction.

The Napoleon type and the Edison type are at the opposite poles, the first being highly negative, self-centred and destructive, the other highly positive, socially useful and constructive, and yet both types lived their dreams in their waking hours.

The drudges, on the other hand, only realize their desires in their sleep and hence need more sleep. Every one knows how sleepy small towns and their inhabitants always appear. People in country towns sleep more than dwellers in large cities although the latter lead a much more active life and hence should require a longer period of rest.

Large cities with their varied life, their exciting bustle, their noise, their accidents, etc., make life, even for the very poor, the overworked and the stupid, a more stimulating set of experiences than the well regulated existence one must lead in a small, settled and uninteresting village.

Monotony seems to be after all the direct cause of sleep. One falls asleep while witnessing a monotonous play, while listening to monotonous music or a monotonous sermon. While noises are supposed to prevent us from sleeping, a very monotonous noise like the tic tac of a metronome or the rumble of a train, can induce very profound and "restful" sleep. In fact a subject who has fallen asleep while concentrating on the beat of a metronome is likely to wake up suddenly when the instrument is stopped. I sleep well in Pullman cars but I invariably wake up when the train stops at a station, although the whispered conversation of other travellers entering the sleeping car and their footsteps muffled by heavy matting are incomparably less noisy than the thundering of a speeding train.

Likewise drunken stupor overtakes the weak and inactive sooner than the strong and active who proceed to satisfy their cravings in their waking state and grow jovial or coarse, if not violent.

Sensitive, dissatisfied people never seem to have enough sleep and escape reality in their waking hours through day dreams which are very similar in every respect to night dreams and during which the subject's anaesthesia is almost as complete as in sleep, the subject being indifferent to many sounds or light stimuli, being as we say, "absent-minded," in a sort of hypnoidal state which does not strike observers as sleep because his eyes remain open.

If we sleep mostly at night it is precisely because

night, on account of the lack of colour, which makes the world more uniform, and the lack of light, which makes motions slower and more difficult, creates the very monotony which induces sleep.

Many experiments have been made on dogs, proving that as soon as their eyes have been closed painlessly, their ears plugged and their legs wrapped in soft rags, the animals fall asleep and remain asleep until exterior stimuli are once more allowed to strike their senses and supply them with the "entertainment" which they probably seek in sleep. For animals dream, as any one who has watched hunting dogs asleep can testify.

That fatigue should enable us to sleep is not an argument in favour of the rest theory but is due to the fact that after over-exercise, our preceptions are not as keen as they were and life is perceived more dully and appears more monotonous. Hence the escape from it through dreams.

The theory of rest through unconsciousness is exploded by the fact that when overtired we cannot sleep. The reason is not far to seek.

When the organism reaches the point of exhaustion, the phenomenon of the second wind takes place. An excessive amount of glycogen comes out of the liver, filling all the muscles with new energy, much as a motorist piloting a weak engine up a hill would "step on the gas," and adrenin creates a tension which seems to make all our sense perceptions infinitely keener (hence the irritability of the very tired person, contrasting strongly with the apathy of the moderately fatigued individual).

In over-exertion the mind becomes unusually alert and often obsessed by one apparently important idea. Hence the lack of monotony and stimulation which otherwise would induce sleep.

Fatigue, we say, is conducive to sleep, but in certain respects, fatigue *is* sleep. For fatigue in its turn is easily induced by very monotonous tasks. The limit of exhaustion is reached more slowly if at all when the occupations are varied and work is performed in a constantly changed environment.

Fatigue is often produced without any physical or mental exertion by a monotonous stimulus. We hear very often people complaining that some one's droning voice "tired them out." Every one of us has had the experience of feeling an uncontrollable desire for sleep when in the company of some extremely dull person whose personality and intelligence radiate absolutely no stimulation.

This view of sleep may throw a little light on the nature and causes of sleeplessness.

Sleeplessness may have physical causes. Overindulgence in coffee, tea or cocoa creates a state of

[194]

anxiety which is not favourable to sound sleep as it makes one more sensitive to stimuli, causes one for instance "to jump" at slight noises and other unexpected happenings.

Lack of physical exercise leaves the body stocked up with energy-producing fuel which we may finally eliminate by tossing about in our bed more or less angrily (anger, by the way, is a good fuel-producing factor leading to more sleeplessness).

Drinking too much water before retiring may compel us to arise several times to urinate. Partaking of laxative fruit or drugs may initiate abdominal activity likely to wake us up, even if no movement is induced.

Overeating and hunger alike create great discomfort unfavourable to peaceful sleep. Heat and cold also can keep one awake. People suffering from cold feet should use a bed warmer; people perspiring freely will perspire even more freely at night and hence should avoid piling up too many blankets on their beds.

In most households beds face a window, which enables the first rays of light to awake the sleeper. Too many husbands and wives share the same bed, thereby disturbing each other's sleep by tossing about or snoring.

[195]

All the physical causes should be removed first and can easily be removed when one is troubled with sleeplessness.

Of the so-called mental causes, worry is the most common and the most distressing. It is perfectly absurd to advise a patient not to worry. When some person dear to us is in danger of death, when one is threatened with a catastrophe of some kind, when some terrible responsibility has to be borne and some weighty problem involving one's future or reputation has to be solved, such advice should be, and generally is, resented. Sleeplessness in such cases is unavoidable but should not be taken tragically, the less so as it is hardly ever unbroken by "cat naps" or spells of almost complete unconsciousness.

People exaggerate greatly their sleeplessness. Experiments made at a Western University when several men were kept forcibly awake for 90 hours showed that on several occasions, when the subjects imagined themselves awake, they had been actually dozing with their eyes open. Their inability to notice certain stimuli showed that for varying periods of time they had not been awake, although they remained in a sitting or standing position. On several occasions too, their answers to questions showed that they had been dreaming.

[196]

Old. people, in particular, tell very unreliable stories about their inability to sleep. As a matter of fact old people whose vagotonic activities are at a very low ebb, need little dream-producing sleep.

Repressed and ungratified desires do not torture the old as they do the young.

Resenting or fearing sleeplessness are undoubtedly the most insidious ways of inducing or prolonging it. As I mentioned before, anger creates a nervous tension and causes the release of energy producing secretions, and so does fear, although to a different degree.

The person who works himself up into a rage because he cannot sleep, and he who retires with his mind full of fear at the possibility of a sleepless night are not likely to "rest" peacefully.

An obsession is easily created: "I am losing my sleep," and it can be used neurotically in an unconscious attempt at obtaining sympathy and shirking some of life's duties. After which, it establishes itself as one of the expedients of the negative life.

Some subjects are unable to sleep on account of their fear of nightmares. This amounts to a stubborn unconscious resistance against some craving which expresses itself symbolically through an anxiety dream. Some of the symbolic dreams I mentioned at the beginning of this chapter will help the reader to understand what I mean. A very puritanical woman might well remain awake to avoid an anxiety dream satisfying her sexual cravings in a symbolical and apparently painful way.

It is evident that when no physical cause can be discovered which would induce sleeplessness, and when no definite worry is keeping the mind (and the liver and adrenals) in a state of activity, there is some recurring dream, forgotten night after night, which the sleepless one is trying to avoid because it expresses some craving subjected to a strong repression.

In both cases, analysis is the only possible means of dealing with the difficulty. The harrowing anxiety dream must be interpreted and the craving it satisfies abnormally, made clear to the sufferer.

In the second case, the unknown complex must be unearthed and the unknown dream traced through day dreams induced in the analyst's office.

Insight into nightmares is easily acquired which soon divests them of their symbolic mask and transforms them into simpler and grosser wish-fulfilment dreams devoid of any anxiety element. A conscious search for the "unknown nightmare" starts an unconscious activity which breaks down the resistance owing to which it is constantly forgotten; after which it can be disintegrated or translated into its actual meaning.

Thousands of recipes for curing sleeplessness have been offered to sufferers, most of them inefficient when not dangerous.

It goes without saying that avoiding all the physical causes of sleeplessness which I listed above should be the first step in any common-sense treatment of that disturbance. But that alone cannot be relied upon to effect a cure when some complex is responsible for the insomnia.

We have all met healthy individuals who manage to sleep like logs in spite of having committed all the possible dietetic indiscretions and of leading the most unreasonable existence. Those are not troubled by any conscious factors.

Staring at, or listening to, a monotonous stimulus may help in many cases. Prayer, recommended by Dr. Thomas Hyslop, by William James and by Dr. Richard C. Cabot, can be considered as such a stimulus; when repeated many times, without emotion and with the automatism which characterizes the delivery of pieces learnt early in childhood, it naturally creates the monotony from which we strive to escape through sleep.

Under no circumstances should narcotics be

[199]

used. They do not produce sleep but a form of unconsciousness akin to death. They are merely poisons taken in too slight a dose to kill us.

Sleep induced by narcotics may not be accompanied by any dreams and is therefore useless. Users of narcotics often complain of terrible nightmares. Such nightmares may not be the gratifying wish-fulfilment dreams which alone make sleep valuable and refreshing.

Sleep should be a display of vagotonic activity in an obvious or symbolic form. Narcotics creating a deep disturbance of the normal life functions, probably occasion in the organism a terrific struggle accompanied by intense organic fear which cannot be beneficial.

BIBLIOGRAPHY

The most useful book to consult on the subject is A. BRUCE's "Sleep and Sleeplessness" (Little, Brown) which epitomises within two hundred pages all the theories of sleep from that of W. H. Hammond to the more recent observations of Marie de Manaceine.

Freud's theory of dreams must be studied with great care, as his large book, "The Interpretation of Dreams," (Macmillan) is not by any means easy to understand at first reading. It might be well for beginners to read first Freud's abbreviated edition of it which is now out of print but can be found in every library.

[200]

CHAPTER II.   SELF-KNOWLEDGE THROUGH DREAM STUDY

Dream study enables us to unravel the mystery of sleep. We sleep that we may dream and, while dreaming, gratify the many cravings which in our waking hours must remain unsatisfied if not severely repressed. Dream study will likewise prove helpful in acquiring that most elusive form of knowledge, knowledge of ourselves.

It is comparatively easy to know others. Our unconscious imitation of their attitudes when we observe them makes us experience in an obscure way the mental and chemical processes of which those attitudes are surface manifestations.

Only in very few cases are the conclusions we draw from our observations of others or which we derive from our unconscious imitation of them, biased by friendship or hostility. In the majority of cases we are probably impartial judges, as impartial at least as our complexes allow us to be.

How difficult it is for us, on the other hand, to judge ourselves.

We may stand before a mirror and try to observe our own attitudes, but as soon as we see our reflection, we involuntarily modify our pose and facial expression and assume others more in harmony with our idealized conception of ourselves. We make infinite allowances for our shortcomings, mental and physical. We refuse to see ourselves as others would see us.

That refusal is simply one of the protective measures life has forced upon us, one of the repressions which in certain cases create bad complexes. The object and subject are too close to each other.

On many occasions we suspect that our unconscious may be thwarting our views of others and we may make an effort at being fair. But we are seldom in doubt as to our opinion of ourselves. And yet how many times do we surprise or grieve ourselves by behaviour for which we can not account satisfactorily.

Some unconscious factor forces our hand at times, we lose control of ourselves, we begin something and suddenly abandon it, we break our promises and suffer remorse and refer to the situation by saying: I don't know what made me do that.

Knowledge of our autonomic tendencies throws light upon the general direction of our unconscious activities, but the information thus gathered is not sufficient to enable us to devise plans for constructive behaviour.

While the Aschner test merely warns us against overdetermination by "nervous" factors, dreams will furnish us with particulars of our unconscious cravings and reveal them to us one after another.

The thing to do then is to collect our night dreams and study them carefully, translating into understandable stories the symbolic pictures which often disguise our night thinking.

But a serious problem has to be solved first: many people forget their dreams completely and boldly assert that they never dream. All of us dream all night long at a terrific speed. Wake up at any time during the night the most "dreamless" sleeper and he will awaken out of a dream. Wake him up by means of some painful stimulus, like a pin prick, and he will tell an extremely long story built around that pin prick in perhaps a couple of seconds.

How shall we then remember some of those numberless dreams?

We must first of all "wish" to remember them. Every wish influences our dreams to a certain extent. Such a wish formulated by an ailing person preoccupied with his health is likely to be a strong

[203]

one and will be more or less completely gratified in his sleep.

This statement will be met with incredulity by many laymen who have not made the attempt. Subject after subject, however, who concentrates on that wish at the time of retiring reports the same experience in almost the same words: I had many dreams that night and during those dreams I was repeating to myself: this is something I must remember so as to tell my analyst.

The first attempts are not all successful. Many subjects simply become conscious of the fact that they dream but remember only scraps of dreams.

Those scraps, however, are valuable and will help in many cases to reconstruct the missing parts of the story.

It may happen also that the subject has, when awaking, a clear memory of several of the night's dreams but proceeds to forget them by the time his eyes are fully open and he is again conscious of his surroundings.

A simple expedient can be used then which will be found very effective. Set the alarm clock an hour ahead of the time at which you usually awaken. Have a pad and pencil ready near your bed and when the alarm rings begin to jot down without arising your dreams, which will then be very fresh and graphic.

Any one, concentrating on dreams before retiring and awaking himself suddenly in the early morning by means of an alarm clock, should within a week train himself to remember very clearly at least one of each night's dreams.

Dreams must be transcribed at once. Our unconscious is both anxious to express itself and afraid of being detected. By five o'clock in the afternoon, the dreams which were so vivid to us on awaking have either dissipated or been "edited." If you write down your dreams in the morning and try to write them down again from memory at night, the discrepancies between the two versions will prove amusing if not distressing.

Those discrepancies should be the first point on which your investigation should bear. "I was walking in the woods with a blonde woman," a patient wrote in his note book immediately on awakening. "I was walking in the woods with some people," he wrote the same night, when rewriting the same dream in accordance with my instructions.

In the course of the day his unconscious had attempted to blur the memory of a woman who

[205]

played in his life a part more important than he was willing to confess even to himself.

The next step in the study of a dream is to take every word of it and to determine its associations. Close your eyes and think of the word or sentence and let your mind use it as a starting point for some short "day dream." Note down whatever ideas are brought forth by that word or sentence, without exercising any critical censorship over the results. The associations may be silly, shameful or merely unpleasant. Honesty in recording them will be, not only a scientific way of collecting material, but a beginning in the training to face facts which every normal or abnormal person, especially the latter, must undergo in order to acquire insight.

Read over the list of associations brought forth by all the words or ideas of the dream until they begin to tell you a story.

Do not, however, expect the first dream or the first ten or twenty dreams to tell you all you wish to know.

This work, slow and tedious, must be kept up day after day, week after week, until you are able to classify your dreams and the various pictures which they present.

Certain dreams will reappear frequently, certain characters will take part in every action presented

[206]

on the dream stage, certain details of scenery will recur night after night, and so will certain situations, emotions, etc.

According to whether the majority of dreams refer to the past, the present or the future they may reveal a regressive, a static or a positive tendency. A neurotic has a tendency to regress to an easier, more protected form of life, symbolized by his childhood. When acquiring insight and improving, he will, in all likelihood, formulate solutions for the problems of the present day in terms of the present day. After recovering he will, in his dreams as in his waking hours, make plans for the future.

It will be found that the "purely obvious" dreams are very scarce and that even those lend themselves to a symbolic interpretation.

The emotional nature of a dream is not a safe guide as to its actual importance. A woman patient dreamt that she was seated in the balcony of an Episcopal church. A man she loved was seated with his wife in one of the pews and looked bored.

The woman was a Christian, the man a Jew and she was extremely jealous of his attentions to his wife. The egotistical desire for domination was strong in her.

The dream, apparently indifferent and unemotional, gratified all her cravings in the following way:

She was seated in the balcony *above her lover and his wife.*

They had come to attend the services in *her church;* that is, they had adopted *her point of view.*

He looked *bored,* hence was *not enjoying his wife's company.*

The character of the building *precluded between man and wife any of the intimacies* to which my patient objected so strongly.

Even as the patient remained unmoved through the dream owing to her inability to understand its meaning or her unconscious resistance to accepting its meaning, others will be extremely agitated by emotion connected with a dream whose horror is not real but only symbolical.

Nightmares, as I stated in the preceding chapter, often melodramatize very simple actions the desire for which we have so repressed that they only break through the repression after an intense struggle. The struggle translates itself into a feeling of horror which is in no way justified or reasonable.

It may be stated that no nightmare has a purely physical cause, such as overeating, bodily discomfort, etc. Thousands of people sleep peacefully after a heavy dinner or in spite of great suffering.

There are many convenience nightmares which endeavour to interpret physical stimuli in a plausible way so that the sleeper will not awake. They spin a story about the pain or discomfort which may be felt and explain it away, so to speak. Others seem to use the actual pain or discomfort as a basis for a horrible presentation which tortures the sleeper and often wakes him up.

Certain nightmares have the value of a warning, for instance in cases of incipient disease which has escaped observation. Heart, stomach or lung disturbances may be revealed by dreams in which those organs play a prominent part. Silberer dreamt several times that a black cat was clawing his throat. Soon after, examination of his throat, made necessary by a severe cold, brought to view a small tumour which necessitated a surgical intervention.

But even in such cases, the choice of dramatic means employed by the unconscious to visualize the cravings depends, not on the nature of the physical stimulus, but on the nature of the cravings and complexes seeking an outlet.

In other words, no nightmare should be dismissed as unimportant for it always has a deep

[209]

meaning, sometimes a twofold one. It reveals a fierce struggle for freedom of something that should be set free if possible and in this respect alone is worthy of serious consideration. While visualizing itself, that struggle may take advantage of some physical condition which in certain cases is unknown to the sufferer and this, too, has to be attended to without delay.

Whenever an organ plays a constant part in nightmares, it should be investigated by a physician as it may constitute in the organism a point of least resistance.

In certain cases thorough examination may be valuable in proving to the subject that certain fears of his are ungrounded. A subject bothered by many dreams of impotence was examined by a specialist and pronounced absolutely normal sexually.

His dreams of impotence which had always been connected with great anxiety were soon after replaced by dreams of normal sexual gratification.

Careful study of a nightmare always causes it to disappear or to lose its painful effect. A nightmare, as I explained in the preceding chapter, is simply a symbolic expression of a wish subjected to a strong repression. When we face reality and confess to ourselves certain cravings whose exist-

[210]

ence we have been trying to deny they no longer assume a symbolic mask in our dreams.

The young woman attacked in dreams by various animals and who forces herself to realize that she is tortured by sexual desires, will in all likelihood dream that her desires are gratified in a normal way. The beasts may reappear but her insight will remain even in her sleep and she will not experience any fear for she will know that "it is only a dream."

A subject of mine anxious to become a public speaker but hampered by various circumstances in the realization of his wishes, dreamt night after night that he stood on the platform and tried to speak but was interrupted by small boys creating a disturbance and, at times, drowning his voice with their shouts.

Analysis of that nightmare proved that his persecutors were conjured up by his unconscious in an egotistical effort to explain away certain deficiencies. Small boys appeared again in the subject's dreams, but they were no longer hostile factors and after a while they disappeared entirely.

Nightmares may be the precursors of a neurosis. Unconscious habits of thought revealed by dreams easily come to dominate our waking thought. A benign neurosis is after all a dream (wish-fulfilment) from which we are trying to awaken ourselves and a pernicious neurosis is a dream from which we do not wish to free ourselves.

Insight into one's mental workings causes them without any exception to become more normal.

When we are fully aware of the childish, regressive character of some of our dreams, they begin to change and to acquire a more positive tenor. A change for the better as well as a change for the worse always appears in the unconscious before it is observable in our conscious states. Even as a nightmare may warn the observer of an oncoming neurotic attack, a positive dream of peaceful accomplishment generally heralds a return to normality.

The results of dream study have many applications to our conscious waking life.

Many family conflicts are due to perfectly unconscious father or mother fixations. A neurotically inclined boy, overattached to his mother, may unconsciously hate his father and *unconsciously* direct all his energies toward defeating all of his father's plans. A neurotically inclined girl, overattached to her father, may also hate her mother unconsciously and conduct *unconsciously* a constant campaign of disparagement against her mother.

Dreams will reveal that situation very soon. The subject, victim of a fixation, will often dream of the favourite parent who appears in complicated

[212]

situations, especially in nightmares, to solve all difficulties. The hated parent will either never appear or be placed in a situation of inferiority. One subject with a father fixation saw her mother in a dream as a drunken beggar. One man with a mother fixation saw his father driving his automobile from a back seat while he sat in the front seat and gave his father directions.

Warned by their dreams of such absurd situations of which they are not conscious, students of dreams can revise their attitudes to members of the family circle. Knowing that certain complexes of a childish character are prejudicing them against some one they can effect a readjustment in their relation to that person.

Dreams not only tell us what we unconsciously think but how we think. The more normal and independent we are, the more obvious our forms of wish-fulfilment are likely to be. Complicated, symbolic dreams should therefore be characteristic of repressed, pent up personalities.

The man with a mother fixation who simply relies upon his mother in dream emergencies is undoubtedly of a less assertive and less carnal type than the one who has the typical Oedipus dream of incest with his mother. The man who either kills his father or attends his father's funeral in a dream

[213]

is very different in his make up from the man who places him in the back seat of an automobile and orders him about.

Also a knowledge, however superficial, of the most common dream symbols may prevent us from worrying about certain dreams of a primitive and childish type, such as the Oedipus dreams.

The man who commits incest or kills his father in dream is not by any means abnormal or perverse and should not consider himself as such. He is simply expressing in a very crude way his affection for one parent and his indifference to the other.

The young mother who dreams of the death of her children may be simply hankering for a little more freedom from household cares and express-ing it in the archaic fashion which our unconscious often affects.

Dream murderers, however, can save themselves from further dream guilt by acquiring insight into the meaning of their sleeping fancies.

Our unconscious dominates our thinking by our leave only. When we set to work to watch our un-conscious it is soon shorn of its harmful power and can become a great power for constructive work.

For almost every one of the cravings revealed by dreams there is some form of positive satisfac-tion. When we seek that satisfaction normally

[214]

our dream work no longer gives it to us in an abnormal form.

Nietzsche spoke truly when he said that we must not seek to dodge the responsibility for our dreams, for nothing, he adds, is more completely the work of our "mind."

BIBLIOGRAPHY

A small book by I. Coriat, "The Meaning of Dreams" (Little, Brown), will prove of great assistance to beginners attempting to analyse their own dreams. A list of the most important symbols can be found in the chapter on "Symbols" of my book on "Psychoanalysis, its History, Theory and Practice."

See also Smith Ely Jelliffe's "The Rôle of Animals in the Unconscious," *Psychoanalytic Review*, No. 3, 1917.

A monograph by K. Abraham, "Dreams and Myths," published by the Nervous and Mental Disease Pub. Co., will reveal to the reader the rather puzzling relations which have been discovered between myths and dream formations.

V. PROBLEMS OF SEX

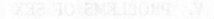

CHAPTER I: THE LOVE LIFE

It is not love in the sense of an affectionate relationship but in the sense of a physical attraction and stimulation which shall be discussed in this chapter. Affection is a very elastic term, in no way dependent upon sexuality. It may exist between master and dog; we may become attached to an old house, a piece of furniture or a suit of clothes, out of habit; for congenial people, we may experience, regardless of their age or sex, a profound feeling in which interest, respect and confidence may blend.

Very different is the attraction which a human being may feel for, or exert upon, another human being of the opposite sex. I might suggest the word erotropism to designate that relation, a word coined on the model of heliotropism, the force which causes certain animals and plants to turn irresistibly toward the sun.

What causes a male or a female to go forth and seek a certain type with which to mate, a type which to others might perhaps appear unattractive, and to disregard entirely many other individuals who, to a third person, might seem infinitely more desirable?

Many sentimental explanations have been ventured by poets and psychologists, but they are, at best, expressions of personal feelings of the most deceptive sort.

Nietzsche, who has written an enormous amount of nonsense on the subject of women but who, in many respects, came "intuitively" to the same conclusions as the various analysts, wrote in 1878, long before Freud began his investigations, this Freudian statement:

"Every one bears within himself an image of woman, inherited from his mother; it determines his attitude toward women, whether to honour them, to despise them or to remain indifferent to them."

The study of the love life of neurotics has enabled psychoanalysts to give a positive answer often formulated in a naïve way: What can she see in him, what can he see in her?

The neurotic only accentuates certain general human traits and tendencies and he makes them, thereby, easier to observe. It is an axiom of psychoanalysis that normal people are labouring under the same unconscious burdens which crush neurotics. Most of us, however, bear the burden without a visible strain; most of us, in other words,

[220]

remain healthy "mentally" as most of us, in spite of our indiscretion in matters of diet, of working and housing conditions, manage to retain our "physical" health.

The neurosis simply acts as a magnifying glass.

In the male neurotic, the choice of a mate is absolutely conditioned by the mother-image, in the female neurotic by the father-image. The neurotic who is absolutely unconscious of his mother fixation, is likely to develop very little interest in any woman, until perhaps his mother dies, when he is likely to marry a woman resembling in many respects his mother as she was when he acquired his fixation, that is between his fifth and his fifteenth years.

If the male neurotic, on the other hand, is partly conscious of his fixation, he may in extreme cases avoid all women, whom he unconsciously identifies with his mother, or in less serious cases, seek a woman who in every possible respect is different from the mother-image.

The same applies to female neurotics affected by a father fixation.

The resemblance between the love-object and the parent-image is at times complete in every respect. It may bear upon one or several physical or mental characteristics or emphasize certain complicated situations. An old maid with a father fixation said to me once. "I have never married because I have never fallen in love with any man who was not married." Her love-object had to have a wife, like her father.

In certain cases the fixation bears rather on attitudes than on physical traits, for it has been observed that the child of a neurotic is likely to seek as his or her mate a neurotic in preference to a normal person.

Experimentation with animals has confirmed the great importance of the mother image in the selection of a mate.

Passenger pigeons have never been known to mate normally with ring doves. But let a ring dove hatch the eggs of a passenger pigeon and the young male passenger pigeons thus brought to life will readily mate with ring doves who represent the mother image; not only that, but they will refuse to mate with female passenger pigeons to which their "heredity" or their "instinct" should draw them, but which are too unlike the mother image.

It is probable that all human beings, like all animals brought up under normal conditions, are guided in their choice of a mate by the father or mother image which has obsessed their consciousness in childhood.

[222]

And this is probably a part of the great secret of the permanency of the species.

This observation enables us to understand the statement often made by laymen that propinquity is the best preparation for love. People who associate constantly and who are not, like brothers and sisters, separated by the incest taboo, may gradually discover in each other a likeness to the parent image which may be too faint to be noticed at first glance. This constitutes a rather good basis for a quiet form of married relationship, for the mere fact that the mates have shared the same environment predisposes them also to a more congenial relationship.

Love at first sight, on the other hand, is the result of a sudden and striking discovery of the parent type by one of the mates or both. This leads easily to uncontrollable outbursts of desire and passion but more rarely to a peaceful life in common.

The parent type may be found in a person who socially, intellectually and morally is not adapted to a certain ideal of family and community life. Nature, however, only considers the race and makes no preparations for intellectual achievements, besides striving to produce the best possible organisms and nervous systems.

The failure of many unions due to such outbursts is not an argument against their biological value.

Marriage being, not an ideal state, but a compromise between what the human animal would like to do and what it can actually do at the present time, in a given state of civilization and culture, has to take into account the reactions of the environment to any phenomenon taking place in that environment.

Family and community peace are better served by a union in which the intellectual agreement will be perfect than by one in which the physical adaptation leaves nothing to be desired. Our associates do not share our sexual life, but they expect to share our social activities, and hence make more demands as far as these are concerned.

It can be easily understood why unions in which one of the mates is a neurotic are not likely to prove very successful. The normal man is "guided" by the mother image in his search for a mate, and he realizes that marriage is a compromise. The neurotic is absolutely "determined" in his selection by an obsessional image and the neurotic temperament is essentially averse to compromises.

The neurotic who has married a woman solely because she corresponded to the mother image, is likely to annoy her whenever she deviates in her speech or conduct from her prototype.

"Mother would do this thing differently,"

[224]

"You should see the way mother would manage this," etc., and many other nagging phrases make up the woof of the neurotic's conversation with his wife.

The wife who has been selected on account of her dissimilarity to the neurotic's mother is perhaps in a worse plight yet. She will be daily taunted for being so different from her husband's mother and we have seen how this sort of treatment accorded to an unfortunate young woman was one of the contributing factors of her severe mental upset.

The desire to dominate one's life partner, a typically neurotic and negative trait, is found to a certain extent in every normal human being. Ardent love is seldom observed unaccompanied by an effort to encroach upon the freedom and personality of the love object.

Jealousy is one of the most common manifestations of the will-to-power in the love life. In the normal man, jealousy is an angry fear of losing something which to the human organism is the strongest stimulus known. The stronger and the more pleasurable the stimulus was the more violent jealousy may be.

In the neurotic type, jealousy contains more anger than fear. The neurotic burdened with a feeling of inferiority resents the fact that one human being, heretofore subjected to his will, is freeing himself from that bondage and subjecting himself to some one else's will. Careful analysis of the neurotic's jealousy shows that the painful element in that emotion is not so much sex as ego. The visualization of the love object in some one else's embrace which, to the normal individual is the most torturing thought, is in the neurotic's mind secondary to the thought of the power which some one else will yield upon the love object.

In fact several forms of pernicious neuroses are characterized at their onset by attacks of absolutely unjustified jealousy, whose absurd or exaggerated form causes the patient to inquire into his own sanity. A patient treated by a well known New York psychiatrist imagined that his wife was deceiving him with a man who entered the house through a door which he knew never existed and which was suddenly opened in a wall which he knew to be absolutely solid.

Apart from the sexual gratification vouchsafed by love, lovers derive many non-sexual forms of comfort from their relationship.

Some of those verge slightly upon a regression to a primitive level. Ardent courtship admitting no third party is a sort of introversion and with-

[226]

drawal from the world, physically and sentimentally, into privacy and romance.

The introversion is quite marked in the conversations of lovers who derive an immense unconscious satisfaction from the fact that they themselves are almost the exclusive topic of conversation. They never tire of telling each other what they think of each other and of themselves and such statements encounter little if any opposition.

The regression appears also in the holding of hands, a childlike gesture symbolizing a craving for reassurance and safety in the parent's keep, and in the baby talk which is not infrequent among lovers.

Infantile caresses and baby talk are quite symbolical of a resumption of life with the mother or father represented by their image in our love mate, of our searching for almost the same comfort we derived as infants and children from our parents.

That apparent regression, however, is neither neurotic nor negative. The constant search for precedents to every action is a negative trait and a factor of stagnation. Constant disregard of precedents, on the other hand, would be destructive and in the field of science a cause for complete and hopeless regression.

Love, being the origin and source of life and the

moulder of the species, has to be conservative if the species is to retain the characters it has acquired in the slow course of evolution.

Another form of pleasure which lovers derive from each other's company may be understood when we recall the experiments made on fishes. If the environment of a living being can exert on that living being such a thoroughgoing modification that colours or objects seen by the eye can be reproduced on the surface of the body, the sight of a loved environment is likely to produce a deep impression on the lover.

And we must bear in mind that the discovery relative to the influence of vision may be supplemented some day by other observations on the influence of our innumerable sense organs, of which new ones are constantly being catalogued.

Herein we may find the explanation of a fact often mentioned by laymen, that a man and a woman, after years of constant association, may grow to look alike; if a fish looking at a pattern on the sides or bottom of its aquarium can, after a lapse of time, reproduce its environment, look like that environment, what difficulty is there in grasping the reason why life mates, after looking at each other for years, reproduce each other's appearance and look alike?

[228]

Scientific literature and fiction alike have emphasized the healthy and buoyant look of the happy lover; fiction in particular has never tired of depicting sympathetically the opposite type, the disappointed lover, pale, feverish, depressed, bereft of his appetite and of all ambition.

Those lists of symptoms are confirmed by a glance, even superficial, at a map of the autonomic nervous system.

Happiness in love means the perfect functioning of the cranial and sacral divisions of the autonomic system, which upbuild the individual and the race, assure a good digestion, regular metabolism, calm and powerful heart beats, the normal elimination of waste matter.

Unhappiness in love or sorrow due to the loss of the love object means a stoppage or reversion of the gastric and intestinal peristalsis, palpitations, constipation, etc.

Study of the autonomic system reveals how closely ego, sex and nutrition activities are related to one another and it is worth while mentioning that the vocabulary of all races reveals that relationship.

The girl we love is "sweet," so sweet we could "eat her up" and "devour" her with kisses; we are "hungry" for her caresses, and confectioners of all nations have some dainty or other which is called "kisses."

The very gestures of the lover are vaguely reminiscent of those made by some marine creatures which throw their tentacles around their victim and after immobilizing it apply their mouths to it and absorb it.

The part played by the parent image in the genesis of love should be recalled when we wish to answer the question: why does love die?

As the love object changes with age, its appearance may not correspond any longer to the parent image which was originally responsible for the erotropism culminating in a permanent union. The organic "reasons" the love subject had for "loving" the love object no longer exist. The white haired and stout wife no longer reminds her husband's unconscious of his blonde and slender mother, nor does the bald and portly husband represent any longer to his wife the father image which captivated her.

And in this connection, I would suggest a more systematic study of a phenomenon designated as fetichism and which in certain cases is the basis of a sexual perversion.

Certain parts of the body wield a stronger physical attraction than others on certain individuals.

[230]

They create memory images of such compelling power that inanimate objects symbolizing them are often cherished greatly by lovers. (A lock of hair may bring back the memory of beautiful tresses, a glove, that of a loved hand.)

Every human being is unavoidably attracted by some part of the love object's body and that part varies with every human being.

Starting with the theory of parent fixation as a basis for attraction we may assume that the part or parts constituting the fixation played a special rôle in the life and activities of the present image.

In its perverse form, fetichism shows the absolute domination of one part of the body or of its symbol, in acute cases being even more potent than the part it represents.

In Mirbeau's novel, "Memoirs of a Chambermaid," we have a pervert, whose sexuality can only be aroused by the sight or feel of women's footwear. The case is taken from real life and is not an unusual one.

All human beings are fetichists to a certain degree and between Mirbeau's neurotic and the young man who gazes fondly at his sweetheart's picture, there is a difference of degree, not of kind.

As a matter of practical conduct it would be most useful to determine the amount of fetichism which enters into the make-up of every case of erotropism. If each mate could determine accurately what parts of his person determined the erotropism of his partner, a conscious effort might be made to retain as completely as possible the part made attractive by fetichism, and thus to prolong the affective duration of the partner's love.

The discarded love object very unjustly charges the lover who has grown indifferent with being fickle, changing, faithless.

The truth is that the victim of that fickleness is the one who has changed, who no longer recalls to his or her mate's unconscious the parent image, and hence cannot any longer determine his or her erotropism.

I might compare the "victim" to a dead battery which no longer produces any current. If the fickle one fails to receive a "thrill" it is not because he is no longer a good conductor but because there is no longer any current he could conduct.

It goes without saying that there are men and women of the so-called "indifferent" type, who are never aroused very deeply because their autonomic system, being perfectly poised, has a tendency to re-establish constantly the balance of the secretions of the vagus system and those of the sympathetic system, together with the emotions and attitudes which correspond to them. That type is eminently suited for the life struggle, as it "recovers" quickly, never remains long under the sway of any emotion and is ready to record new emotions, accurately but briefly. Such people do not remain in love very long and are likely to be berated soundly for their coldness.

The reproaches addressed to them are both just and unjust: they are built organically so as to resist a too complete subjugation by any love object and their attitude is unconsciously determined. On the other hand in the case of a union which should be permanent, they could, by using their will power, place themselves in mental and physical attitudes representing, dramatizing, so to speak, the feelings they wish to experience. A good actor, representing a certain feeling on the stage, causes the audience to experience that feeling for a certain time. We can, by acting certain feelings, produce in ourselves the secretions which correspond to them.

Attitudes can be acquired and, in the case of marriage relations, when complete submission to our unconscious urges is asocial and cruel, a simple rule of behaviour can be offered.

As will power on the other hand is probably the resultant effect of a keen awareness of the various possible choices and of a perfect understanding of their consequences, that assumption of a beneficial attitude is not within every one's reach. And in this case, as in many others, praise or vituperation is out of place.

This must be always remembered when we deal for instance with love's perversions. The word perversion is generally fraught in the layman's mind with loathsome connotations.

A perversion is, to many, due to "low," "animal," "filthy," "criminal" instincts. Perversions may be filthy and appear low and animal, but there is nothing "criminal" nor "instinctive" about them. The pervert certainly does not wish to break any law, nor is he impelled by an "instinct." He is a pitiable type whose education and training has made him the imperfect human specimen he is.

Psychoanalysts are all agreed on the genesis of passive male homosexualism. The passive male homosexual is in every case the son of a widow or divorced mother, separated from her husband by death, desertion or legal proceedings soon after the boy's birth.

The boy, compelled to imitate some one in order to have a standard of behaviour, copies his mother's attitude of physical indifference to women and physical interest in men.

In every respect but in the anatomical respect

[234]

he becomes a woman, and later in life will conceive of sexual gratification as woman would. Possession by a man will become his love goal.

Experiments made on pigeons show that the process is the same among those birds. A young male pigeon raised among males in the absence of any female will, when reaching adulthood, be attracted by males only whom he will treat at mating time as though they were females. A male pigeon raised among females only will at mating time play the part of a female.

A pigeon raised in complete isolation from any males or females will try to mate with any inanimate object found in his cage, or with the hand of the person feeding him, and if placed in a cage with a female will pay absolutely no attention to her at mating time.

Here as in the case of passenger pigeons mating with ring doves, instinct proves to be at times infinitely weaker than training.

The study and treatment of sexual perversions are still in their infancy. Men and women practising their perversions are deriving therefrom a minimum of gratification which generally saves them from a well-marked form of neurosis and hence they do not seek the advice of a psychologist. Those who repress their desire for abnormal intercourse and merge into a neurosis are dangerous patients to handle, for they suffer from many delusions of invariably the same content: that is that they receive sexual advances from people of their own sex. Those delusions are likely to apply to the psychiatrist handling their case and unless they are confined in an institution, may very easily start a train of gossip likely to wreck their adviser's reputation.

The perversions known as sadism and masochism, the first being a craving to inflict suffering upon human beings, the latter a craving to torture ourselves or to suffer pain at the hands of another person, may be due in their mild form to the child's lack of understanding of the relationship existing between, for instance, a strong, athletic father and a delicate, slight mother. The playful imitations of violence, the playful and contented pretence at suffering indulged in by the man and the woman when fondling each other in their children's presence, may lead one child to commit in reality cruelties which his father only shammed, another child to seek suffering which his mother seemed to feel.

Acute cases, when a man or a woman experiences no sexual gratification unless they can inflict suffering on their mate or be subjected by their mate

[236]

to cruel treatment, are justly attributed by Freud to the witnessing by young children of their parents' embracing, who misunderstanding the nature of the act identify themselves either with the apparently cruel father or the apparently abused mother.

Like all other maladjustments, the various maladjustments of the love life, perverse or not, call, not for censure or punishment but for understanding and psychological treatment. When for instance the nature of homosexualism, its involuntary character and the fact that it is forced on the "pervert" by his wrong training, and not acquired by him for purposes of gratification, is better known to the general public, psychiatrists and analysts may be able to effect many cures of that "perversion" as well as of sadism and masochism.

BIBLIOGRAPHY

The basis for the theories of love advanced by the various analysts is Freud's "Three Contributions to the Theory of Sex" (Nervous and Mental Disease Pub. Co.) in which he discusses infantile sexuality, puberty and sexual perversions. His discussion of homosexualism in "Leonardo da Vinci" is the least scientific or convincing work of his on the subject. Poul Bjerre, the Scandinavian analyst, presents in his "Theory and Practice of Psychoanalysis" (Badger), several cases illustrating forms of attachment with a morbid complexion. Jacques

Loeb's remarks on Heliotropism in his "Forced Movements, Tropism and Animal Conduct" will supply the reader with several examples of chemical determinism. Perversions are discussed fully in S. Ferenczi's "Contributions to Psychoanalysis."

CHAPTER II: CAN WE SUBLIMATE OUR CRAVINGS?

None of the words created by Freud has lent itself to more misinterpretation than the word *sublimation*. Sublimation is an unfortunate expression. It is not related in its analytic meaning to sublimation as understood by chemists. It becomes involuntarily associated with the adjective sublime and this association is the cause of a good deal of mischief.

By sublimation, Freud understands a process which seeks to utilize the sexual energy, immobilized by repressions and set free by analysis, for higher purposes of a non-sexual nature.

This is of course extremely vague and slightly fantastic and reminds us of the attempts made by alchemists in the middle ages to transmute "base metals" into gold.

We must beware of false analogies: heat can be transformed into power, power into heat and both into light, which in its turn can be transformed into power or heat, but human energy and *energy* as defined by physicists, while probably very similar, cannot be considered as synonymous and treated as such.

The human body is, as Kempf has said, a biological machine, but biological machines and ordinary machinery present one capital difference. While some mechanical apparatus may be so constructed that it can be utilized in ten or twenty different ways at the same time, the use or non-use of one or several of its parts does not affect the other parts. In the human organism all the parts are closely related and abuse or disuse of one of them has a repercussion in all the organs of the body.

A part of a machine may never be used and yet remain in perfect condition if protected against rust. Any part of the biological machine will wither and degenerate unless it is allowed to perform its specific functions. Atrophied muscles and ankylosed joints are the result of lack of normal activity.

Cravings, some people will say, are not to be compared to the play of muscles or joints. The tendency of modern psychology, however, is to identify more and more closely cravings with certain definite segments of the autonomic nervous system, and when that identification has been completed it will be obvious that to the atrophy of a certain nerve there must correspond the atrophy of the craving that nerve carries.

While sublimation is a new word, attempts at sublimation are nothing new. The ascetics who scourged their flesh to kill their "animal" desires, who withdrew into the desert to shun all temptations, were attempting to sublimate their cravings.

In too many cases, the result was not especially gratifying. The repression of a normal craving often meant the appearance of an abnormal symptom. The devil tempted sorely the holy men and women who were fighting the flesh, which meant that they exchanged normal reality for hallucinations, normal desires for perverse desires.

No normal craving can be normally repressed. Nor can it be normally sublimated. Sexual desire cannot be *transformed* into artistic achievement, philanthropy, social usefulness.

Sexual desire may be killed by castration, after which it may be that more energy can be expended by the subject on attaining other goals of a "higher, non-sexual character." Even this is rather dubious, as sexual activity is always linked and almost synonymous with many other organic activities.

The desirability of *sublimation,* except as a social convenience, remains to be proved. Freud's assertion that culture owes many of its conquests to the

sublimation of sexual cravings is contradicted by
the biography of many famous men; let us only
mention Goethe and Rodin, who displayed a feverish creative activity while indulging freely and
openly their sexual desires. Freud attempts to tell
us that Leonardo da Vinci's creative powers may
have been enhanced by his lack of desire for
women's love. But Leonardo was a homosexual
and satisfied his cravings abnormally, which used
up at least as much energy as though he had satisfied them normally.

While guilty of vagueness when propounding his
theory of sublimation, Freud should not be held
responsible for some of the vagaries which some of
his followers and some of the Swiss analysts have
indulged in regarding the desirability and possibility of *sublimating* sexual cravings.

"We must not forget," Freud said in one of his
lectures, "that a part of the suppressed sexual cravings has a right to direct satisfaction and should
find it in life. Exaggerated sexual repression
simply hastens our flight from reality and into a
neurosis without assuring any cultural gain.

"We must not neglect the animal part of our
nature. The elasticity of sex may lure some of us
to attempt a more and more complete sublimation
destined to promote high cultural aims. But even
[242]

as our modern machines can only transform a part of the heat applied to them into useful mechanical work, sublimation can only use for other aims a part of the sexual energy.

"If the repression of sexuality is pushed too far it amounts to a robbery committed against the organism."

And he concluded his lecture with a story which left no doubt as to his opinion in the matter.

A village community kept a horse that could do an enormous amount of work. The wiseacres of the community thought, however, that he consumed too much fodder. They decided, therefore, to train him to subsist on smaller and smaller rations of fodder. The horse was apparently none the worse for his scanty diet. He finally was able to subsist on one stalk of hay a day. The next day, he was to be put to work without any fodder at all. On the morning of that day, however, he was found dead in his stall. The *sublimation* of his craving for food was complete.

The constantly increasing repression to which sexual cravings are submitted, owing to the growing complexity of community life, compel every thinking human being to give the subject the earnest consideration it deserves.

A mere denial of the possibility of sublimation

[243]

as understood by Freud or a convenient assertion of its possibility by well meaning, though irresponsible moral zealots, will not solve the problem.

The problem, however, has not been formulated properly.

The question is not as to whether we can sublimate the sexual craving as understood biologically, but as to whether we can sublimate the sexual craving as complicated by modern civilization.

Sexual desire at the present day has been completely exiled from polite society, from conversation, from literature, from pictorial representation, and relegated to the bedroom.

Many of its more or less unavoidable consequences, love, affection, tenderness, admiration, etc., have been given an undue prominence for the purpose of drawing a veil over the gross physical phenomena of sex.

As we are too often the victims of the vocabulary we use, many rely upon the vocabulary of polite society to assist them in their flight from gross reality.

A woman unable to voice publicly her desire for sexual gratification declares that she seeks a companion. And she probably means that, too. And if her lack of gratification should be the cause of a neurosis, it would be most important to know

[244]

that her sexual craving is complicated by a craving for companionship.

Almost any craving can be easily gratified in our modern world so long as it remains dissociated from other cravings. The sexual craving being frowned upon by our hypocritical civilization, is constantly associated with many other cravings which the normal man, as well as the neurotic, imagine to be inseparable components of "love."

The love of an individual for an individual of the opposite sex may, according to temperaments, include one or all of the following cravings: domination, companionship, protection, pride, boastfulness, submission, praise, possession of beauty, active or passive tenderness, wealth, romance, excitement.

While every one of these non-sexual cravings may be invoked by men and women to justify sexual indiscretions to which their gratification has led, it may be also stated that in thousands of cases, the sexual gratification was an incident of the gratification of one or several of these cravings.

Flaubert's silly and touching heroine, Madame Bovary, was anything but an oversexed woman carried away by her sensuality. Love, to her, meant romance, sentimental companionship, the translation into real life of the fiction and poetry she had read or memorized, mysterious trysts, perilous situations, obstacles successfully surmounted, the breaking away from conventionality and monotony, an opportunity to give vent to the trashy lyricism which filled her day dreams, etc. Those were really the things she craved but her lack of intelligence, of ability in any direction, of psychological insight, of altruistic guidance, conspired to convince her that in love only could she attain the gratification of all her desires.

When reality proved cruelly deceptive and she saw all her dreams shattered, she fled from reality by the path of suicide.

Others adopt the path of the neurosis, seeking an abnormal gratification of a sometimes very painful type or imagining that all their wishes have been fulfilled and living the unreal life of the insane.

It goes without saying that even a moderate sexuality reinforced and complicated by so many sentimental associations becomes a tyrant against whose domination the subject's will can hardly prevail.

The task of the analyst in such cases is easily defined, although difficult of execution, for the truth in such matters is not always readily ascertained.

While a subject may deny vehemently to his associates that he is obsessed by sexual thoughts, he may in the seclusion of a physician's or an analyst's office, greatly exaggerate those cravings which he aims to make responsible for his condition.

The analyst must then determine all the parasitic elements which have attached themselves to the sexual cravings as barnacles attach themselves to a ship and endeavour to make the subject see them, not as essential details of his obsession, but as separate entities.

Every one of Emma Bovary's cravings could have been satisfied separately in non-sexual ways if she had not relied upon an ideal lover to bring to her all the elements of happiness, if she had entered the road of positive personal achievement.

Likewise many a woman suffering from sick headaches because her husband or lover neglects her and fails to help her carry out her dreams of domination, could be relieved of her symptoms if she could be made to see in how many other directions her will-to-power could exert itself.

After positive means have been agreed upon between the subject and the analyst for the gratification of the various parasitic cravings which have been separated from his sexual craving, there will be a residuum of pure sexuality for which no sublimation can be suggested.

If that craving does not receive satisfaction of

a normal nature it will proceed to satisfy itself in more or less abnormal ways, the least abnormal of which will be, according to the subject's repressions, gross sexual dreams or symbolical anxiety dreams. Further analysis should endeavour to transform such anxiety dreams into obvious dreams so as to avoid the organic waste corresponding to anxiety.

No "ethical" solution, however, can be offered by any honest analyst for the subject who, owing to certain complications of modern life, cannot secure normal sexual gratification.

Religious meditation may satisfy the mystical cravings which are often associated with sexual desire, but it does not satisfy that desire except in abnormal ways, as in the case of Zinzendorf, who imagined himself a woman in the arms of the Heavenly Bridegroom.

Charitable or social work of the philanthropic type will use up the masochistic love components which cause the subject to expend care or tenderness upon others.

Artistic endeavour would gratify egotistical cravings, and so would public speaking, acting, and other activities more or less exhibitionistic in their character.

Joining clubs, societies, etc. is the best way to

satisfy the desire for companionship; organizing new groups and assuming their leadership would relieve the feeling of inferiority which drives one to secure some form of domination.

A thousand other suggestions for craving-gratification of a positive, socially useful and beneficial type can be suggested by the analyst to his subject and should be suggested, but I repeat, none of them will reduce the power of the sexual craving itself.

The sexual craving, however, after being freed of all parasitical cravings, will appear infinitely less insistent.

A comparison with another physical craving will make the point clearer. Certain neurotics are tortured by a constant need to urinate which may be designated as "nervous," for its satisfaction reveals that an insignificant amount of urine has accumulated and that the pressure exerted by it is not sufficient to demand the voiding of the bladder.

It is not the quantity of urine present in the bladder, nor the condition of the bladder or of the urinary passages which creates the need, but some compulsion which uses the urinary organs as a convenient means of self-expression.

When the obsessive ideas connected with urination are removed by analysis, urine can be retained in the bladder for several hours without causing any

[249]

discomfort. In this case we have a parasitic craving attaching itself to a physical function and
making the performance of that function a constantly reappearing need.

Cravings for certain foods disappear, leaving
simply a healthy appetite for those foods, when
the associations which make such foods absolutely
necessary for the subject's peace of mind or happiness have been made conscious. A patient unable to digest anything but milk and hard brown
rolls which he carried in his pocket and constantly
toyed with, began to assimilate easily other aliments when he realized his regression to an infantile diet and to a symbolic form of coprophilism.

His liking for milk and rolls did not pass away
when he gained insight into the unconscious reasons
for his abnormal craving for them. He still considered them as pleasant forms of nourishment but
he was no longer obsessed by the thought of them.

Whether the sexual craving is conscious or unconscious, it should be submitted to a careful analysis leading to its disintegration into a genuine sexual
need and various parasitic cravings.

Finally a word should be said about subjects
who, owing to certain fears, fear of disease, fear
of impotence, fear of "injuring their brain," shun
sexual gratification.

[250]

Their case is generally rather complicated, for their fear itself is a neurotic fancy which leads them to submit to a deprivation likely, in its turn, to cause more neurotic complications.

After their phobia has been analysed and removed, they should be enlightened sexually and freed from the various superstitious beliefs relative to sexual activities which are being spread abroad by quacks or ignorant puritans and upon which the neurotic imagination seizes as a convenient excuse for certain forms of negativism.

BIBLIOGRAPHY

Very little has been published on the subject of sublimation besides Freud's remarks in his lectures on the "Origin and Development of Psychoanalysis," delivered at Clark University. O. Pfister, a lay analyst, of Switzerland, has devoted to it several pages of his book "The Psychoanalytic Method" (Moffat, Yard). "Sanity in Sex" by W. J. Fielding (Dodd, Mead) will offer valuable suggestions to the student of sex problems.

CHAPTER III. PURITANISM A DIGNIFIED NEUROSIS

Humorists very often express in a few lines what long-drawn psychological treatises based on many tests and experiments do not always make very clear. No better analysis of puritanism could be found than that contained in this rather ancient but very pointed story:

A puritanical woman telephoned to the police asking that small boys who were bathing naked in front of her house be arrested. An officer was sent to drive them a mile or so farther down the river.

A few minutes later she called up again: "I can still see them from the roof of the house." Once more a policeman went forth to frighten the urchins away.

Half an hour later, the police station phone rang again: "I can still see them," the puritanical woman said, "through my field glasses."

In other words, a subject, sexually hypersensitive, discovers a sexual stimulus in an object which in a normal subject would not produce any stimulation of a sexual type. The subject resents

[252]

the disturbance thus produced in his sexual life and, unable to resist the attraction of the stimulus, demands that the stimulus be removed by legal intervention.

The records of the New Haven courts dating back to the early days of the New England colonies present that picture over and over again. Many are the cases in which a whole community spied day and night for weeks or months upon some indiscrete pair of lovers and, after satisfying its voyeur instincts, finally delivered them to justice to be whipped for their sins.

The normal indignation of the witnesses was inextricably mixed with a sense of perverse gratification and resentment not entirely devoid of envy.

The puritan, taking the word in its modern acception, is a sexually abnormal person. According to whether its abnormality is anaesthesia or hyperaesthesia, we have two types, both negative socially, one of which, however, is seldom objectionable.

The sexually frigid person whose frigidity is organic, being due to undeveloped genitals or low vitality, cannot understand the influence exerted on normal individuals by sexual stimuli. That type links sexual activities with urinary or anal

[253]

functions and for reasons of delicacy avoids any mention of them.

Such people lead what is generally considered as a "pure" life; suggestive literature, theatrical performances, pictorial art, etc., do not appeal to them, and they are likely to regard any one indulging in sexual pleasure as "low" or "animal."

They have their counterpart in every walk of life, where we meet people who do not care for cabbage, who do not smoke, who do not like to climb mountains and never go fishing, but who at the same time let others eat cabbage, smoke, climb mountains and go fishing.

The hyperaesthetic puritan, on the other hand, is not satisfied with abstaining from cabbage. He wishes to suppress cabbage wherever found and to jail those selling it and eating it.

Oversexed neurotics not only are profoundly disturbed by sexual thoughts and facts but place a sexual complexion on almost everything.

It was only last summer that a Massachusetts woman had her neighbour arrested for allowing his two infants to bathe in the sea without bathing suits. Every summer the sight of one-piece bathing suits for men produces a "brainstorm" in some oversensitive neurotic and bathers are fined by stupid judges. A few months ago a society was formed in New York City to prevent owners of department stores from showing "suggestive" lingerie in their windows.

When we remember that ten years ago or so, the New York Society for the Suppression of Vice raided a perfectly legitimate art school and seized a catalogue containing reproductions of nude drawings made by the pupils of that school, that the same society has caused purely medical books to be excluded from the mails and is at present trying to censor articles appearing in medical publications, we must come to the conclusion that "organized puritanism" is not a constructive force but a neurotic symptom unjustly dignified by the police and the courts, a mere form of sexual hyperaesthesia.

Even the sacred books can furnish those neurotics with sexual stimulation. George Francis Train was jailed in the eighties for publishing the Bible serially in the *Citizen* and thus "debauching the young." . . . A group of puritans investigated Chicago's "vice" a few years ago and drew a sensational report of their findings. Thereupon another group of puritans found that report too fascinating and managed to have it excluded from the mails on the ground of obscenity.

The complexity of modern society makes a great

[255]

amount of sexual repression unavoidable and children, for instance, reaching the age of puberty must be protected against certain dangers. Sexual truths, however, would be a better protection for them than sexual lies, and while puritans usually harp on the protection needed by immature minds, they never make any positive suggestion for making minds more mature.

The puritan himself is extremely immature and romantic. In all puritanical ways of thought-expression we find a large measure of sexual romance.

Scientific terms place upon human intelligence limits beyond which it must not go if it wishes to remain accurate. The words syphilis and gonorrhea not only present definite clinical pictures but strip the diseases they indicate of any romance.

The puritan, on the other hand, who designates them as "social diseases" or "diseases of vice" and fails to describe any of their symptoms, makes them mysterious and hence to certain minds infinitely attractive.

The word pregnancy is generally heard in respectful silence. The expression "an interesting condition" generally elicits a smile.

Likewise, the puritan shuns the words brothel, prostitute, sex, and prefers the more elastic and more suggestive expressions: house of ill fame,

[256]

woman of questionable reputation, animal instincts.

Not only do we find in the puritan vocabulary the vagueness which promotes sexual dreaming but we observe also the inaccuracy and displacement which are characteristic of the neurotic escape from reality. Arms, even bare, are decent, but legs are tolerable only when renamed limbs, the belly becomes the stomach and a woman carries her unborn child "under her heart."

The puritan continually indulges in the disparagement of woman which is one of the most characteristic neurotic and negativist traits. The fear of the sexual partner is intense in the anaesthetic and hyperaesthetic alike. The undersexed is made through intercourse to realize his inferiority, the oversexed is loath to be dominated by his desire. Hence both resent woman and her attraction. The fear of woman, the impure, the temptress, fills the literature of puritanism.

A puritanical judge defined obscenity as "whatever might arouse a libidinous passion in the mind of a modest woman." John S. Sumner said of Dreiser's "The Genius," that he looked at it "from the standpoint of its harmful effects on female readers of immature minds."

The Rev. John Roach Straton discussing spiritualism stated that women are the associates of the devil, constantly in league with him to lead men to perdition and adduced as evidence the fact that the majority of mediums are women.

The puritan is not satisfied with suppressing obvious "evils"; he must uncover hidden evils and, at times, his eagerness to catch sinners gives the impression that he is somewhat of a voyeur.

Clergymen who could not as such attend "suggestive" shows, drink in "gin mills," consort with cabaret dancers or enter "houses of ill repute," can indulge in all those diversions provided they assume the character of moral crusaders.

The next day they gratify their sadism by denouncing and hauling into court the sinners they previously befriended.

In all sexual relations there is a survival of a primitive craving which drives one of the sexual partners to overpower the other. In mammals it is generally the male who overpowers the female. Civilization has repressed that craving in a large degree.

In neurotics, however, a regression takes place which enables the male to avenge himself, so to speak, upon the female, for her domination, by brutalizing her. It generally stops at disparagement, nagging or hatred, but in certain pervert cases there is actual violence offered. The savage persecution of prostitutes by vice-fighters (on one occasion driving them out of their houses and on the streets, without providing any shelter or planning any measures of rescue), points to primitive, barbaric savagery gratifying itself in a cowardly, neurotic way.

I say cowardly because such exhibitions of violence are always countenanced by the mob. Millions of inferior persons without any ability in any direction, lacking in the self-assertion which wealth might give them, unable to force their way into "exclusive circles," are prone to don the mantle of moral righteousness in order to acquire without physical or mental exertion some form of superiority.

Neurotic egotism is strong in puritans who are not satisfied with saving the world from a thousand imaginary dangers but use all the channels of publicity to proclaim their achievements.

Many of those traits were exemplified by Anthony Comstock's life and activities, as described by his official biographer C. G. Trumbull. He was the son of a rather brutal father who added to his cruelty a decided refinement of the perverse sort, sending the lad into the woods to cut the switches with which he was to beat him. Little

[259]

Anthony was in the habit of nicking those switches so that they would break when his torturer applied them too energetically. The reasons for those beatings are not mentioned but another paragraph of the official biography enables us to venture a guess.

"Certain things that were brought into his life in those boyhood days started *memories and lines of temptation that were harder for him to overcome* than anything that ever came into his life in later years."

"He knows what an awful and lasting poison is the poison of impurity. Once gaining entry into a life, through book or story or picture, it stays. . . . There the images stay to be called up freely and used at will by the Devil."

In other words he probably remained all his life the inflammable boy every human being is at the time of puberty and having lingered at that child-like level, was convinced that all mankind was as undeveloped, as easily tortured by temptation as he was, and exposed to all the dangers which frighten the hypererotic.

Fanaticism appeared in his behaviour at an early age. At eighteen he broke into a saloon and spilled all the "liquor" in the place. When he enlisted he would not only refuse to drink his ration

[260]

of whiskey but throw it out on the ground in the presence of his fellow soldiers.

Mustered out from the army he became a dry goods clerk in New York City. He seems to have suffered at that time from the delusions and hallucinations which are frequently observed in the sexually abnormal who repress their cravings through a severe struggle.

"During those six years of varied business experience," his biographer writes, "he had come to know young business men, over and over again, whose lives were plainly *ruined by their interest in the obscene pictures and literature* and other devilish things that they had easy access to. . . . In his close contact with the young business men of the city, he saw them *falling about him almost like autumn leaves,* withered at the blighting touch of the obscenities that were the staple of so much commercialized traffic."

Every analyst has met the syphilophobiac who attributes everybody's sickness, misfortune or death to venereal disease, or the unconscious homosexual who in every gesture which another man makes, sees an improper advance.

Comstock's megalomania revealed itself in his constant reiteration of his belief that God was guiding every one of his actions; he even had auditory hallucinations in which a voice told him where to go to find obscene objects.

In other words, a pitiable type, fit to be treated by psychiatrists and not to be entrusted with the censorship of a nation's morals.

The society he founded displays on every occasion the neurotic craving for power which only annoys but never helps, which punishes but never offers a constructive suggestion for reclaiming culprits.

The desire for suprahuman powers, for the acquisition of a privileged situation in the community has always characterized sexual puritanism from its beginnings. In ancient religions, men or women mentally upset by sexual privation, priests and priestesses of various cults, were credited with superhuman wisdom and their hysterical ravings called oracles.

Several religions have imposed celibacy upon their priests in the belief that such a condition would enable them to rise to a higher spiritual plane. When certain churches began to lose their intellectual leadership they established puritanical restrictions in order to conquer some form of moral leadership.

In our days this procedure is very evident in the antics of a Billy Sunday or a John Roach Straton who, lacking totally in any ideas, resort to vituperation and lavish anathemas on "sinners." If those neurotics could not rise in indignation at the thought of the low gowns and silk stockings worn by young women they would have to remain silent.

It goes without saying that the alliance of puritanism with religion is looked on favourably by those who prefer to see the masses interest themselves in a future life. The exploiter of labour and the profiteer approve of Christianlike resignation and of the acceptance of our trials on this earth.

Thus puritanism secures the support of all the large business interests and becomes well nigh irresistible.

The shallow point of view of organized puritanism is revealed clearly in a letter from John S. Sumner to the writer, dated April 9, 1920. "The influence exerted by such publications, many moving pictures and many dramatic productions, directly harmfully affects family relations and the home which is the basis of our social order. We feel, therefore, that we are doing a fundamental service in seeking to suppress those things which would destroy the basis of our social order."

At a time when unpardonable increases in rentals, in the cost of food and clothing are making it impossible for family men to retain their homes, Mr. Sumner boasts of protecting them against vicious publications, lewd shows and movies. Sexual obsession could not be confessed more frankly.

Puritanism, be it of the undersexed or of the oversexed sort, kills all art manifestations. Art is expression, not repression, and curiously enough, even some of the freer minds among the art critics are yielding to the puritanical pressure and, now and then, praise an actor, a painter or a sculptor for his "power of repression."

Not only the pictorial arts and literature have been stifled in puritan-ridden lands but music even has been neglected.

Remember the absurd statements may by Tolstoy, who was tortured by sexual obsessions and discovered lewdness even in Beethoven's compositions. Few conductors and even fewer orchestra musicians hail from puritan lands. Whatever symphonic compositions such lands have produced could be all ignored in a survey of the world's musical achievements.

Puritans, however, are looking forward to conquests in new territories, some of which had never before been invaded by lay authorities.

The March, 1920, issue of the report of the New York Society for the Suppression of Vice contains two especially distressing items: an announcement that a medical publication has submitted an article for revision by the society; this would indicate that unless powerful opposition is raised against such attempts, science is to become "bowdlerized," which probably means that at some future time venereal clinics will be abolished and operations on the abdomen re-christened operations on the stomach.

Finally the society having hauled into court some offender who was let off with a suspended sentence, *"warned the offender to leave town."*

This is destructive persecution of the worst type, lacking in social intelligence, dumping perverts or criminals upon other communities, getting rid of a disease by trying to let the neighbour catch it, as savages, with the help of witches, are wont to do.

The puritan neurosis will probably pass away when the forces which support it have been fettered and made harmless and when the forces which carry out its decrees, courts and police, having been reformed, will no longer need to hide their moral and ethical inferiority under the mask of sexual austerity.

BIBLIOGRAPHY

The official biography of Anthony Comstock "Anthony Comstock, Fighter," by C. G. Trumbull (Fleming, Revell) is the best source of information as to the workings of the puritanical mind. T. Schroeder in his "Free Press Anthology," C. Pollock in the *Bulletin* of the Authors' League of America for March, 1917, H. L. Mencken in his "A Book of Prefaces" (Alfred A. Knoff), and Frank Harris in *Pearson's Magazine* for June, 1917, cite innumerable cases of puritanical suppression of free thought and free expression in literature and art. Also consult the Monthly Report of the New York Society for the Suppression of Vice which is a record of the "lawful" activities of the organized puritans.

VI. THE PSYCHOANALYTIC TREATMENT

CHAPTER I. HYPNOTIST AND ANALYST

"I suppose suggestion plays a great part in the psychoanalytic treatment," is a statement which every analyst hears frequently and has to deny emphatically. Hypnotism and psychoanalysis not only have nothing in common but are in fact the exact opposite of each other: hypnotism introduces something into the subject's mind, psychoanalysis takes something out of it.

The hypnotist takes certain ready-made ideas, generally considered as ethical or practical, and, taking chances with their acceptability, tries to make the subject accept them because they are likely to be beneficial to him.

The psychoanalyst, having slowly and carefully amassed evidence as to certain ideas which are obsessing the subject and are likely to wreck his health, proceeds to disintegrate them and helps the subject to eliminate them.

The charge often made by ill-informed opponents of psychoanalysis, among them Boris Sidis, that people may be wrecked and perverted by the sexual thoughts suggested in the course of an analysis, reveals a profound ignorance of the psychoanalytic procedure.

The Freudian school is the only one to lay much emphasis on the sexual element, but the orthodox Freudian is an almost extinct species. Even he, however, should be cleared of every suspicion of sexual suggestion. The sexual material is present in every subject, normal or abnormal, and comes to the surface very easily. No suggestion is necessary to bring it forth.

The Freudians consider sex as the all-important factor in the neurosis. The other schools are inclined to seek, behind the sexual mask, other factors assuming a sexual complexion for abnormal reasons. Adler has stated many times that imaginary sexuality deceives the subject but should not deceive the analyst. If an analyst of the Adlerian school ever tried to suggest anything to his subjects it would be the belief that sex is not always sex.

But no analyst ever suggests anything. As we shall see at the end of this chapter, as soon as the rapport between analyst and subject is such that the subject is too easily influenced by the analyst, the analysis is likely to prove a failure.

One of the reasons for the widely spread belief that hypnotism and psychoanalysis are related

[270]

methods of treatment is the fact that several of the best-known analysts originally practised hypnotism.

It was while studying a patient in hypnotic "trances" that Freud suspected the possibility of a study of the unconscious in the waking state. Freud made a deep study of hypnotism under men like Charcot of the Salpétrière and Bernheim and Liébault of Nancy. He soon realized, however, the shortcomings of the hypnotic method and discarded it entirely.

Jung, of Zurich, was discouraged from using hynotism by the brilliant and spurious successes he achieved through it. An old woman among others who would call at his office complaining of some excruciating pains, fall asleep in three seconds and before he had time to even suggest anything, wake up, thank him and go away, convinced him that the hypnotist is simply aiding and abetting an unconscious fraud.

It may be, however, that if Freud, Jung, Ferenczi and the many others who started in life as hypnotists and, after a while, became psychoanalysts, had not become familiar with the psychology of suggested sleep, they would have been at pains to understand the mechanism of certain neuroses.

All students of psychoanalysis should glance at

[271]

a few books on hypnotism for that very reason. It would enable them to convince themselves of the neurotic character of that practice.

There are, briefly speaking, three methods of hypnotizing people: A man of powerful physique and of impressive appearance often succeeds in hypnotizing subjects by ordering them in a stern voice to fall asleep. This method is especially effective with weak, timid, feminine subjects. Some memory of the father's authority is evidently at work in such cases and compels obedience.

Other subjects can only be prevailed to enter the hypnotic state in a quiet, dimly lighted room, when the hypnotist keeps up a flow of soothing, monotonous, often senseless words, spoken in a low, crooning voice and strokes the face and hands of the subject. This is the method employed by every mother singing her infant to sleep and surrounding him with a peace and monotony symbolical of absolute security.

Nervous fatigue is relied upon in other cases to induce artificial sleep, the subject being asked to concentrate his gaze on a brilliant object, such as a diamond held in one position or moved about, or to listen to the ticking of a watch, etc.

Between ten and twenty per cent. of all the subjects examined have been found impossible to hypnotize. No conclusion should be drawn from that condition as to their normality. They may be so normal and independent that the idea of submitting to any one else's will is repellent to them. They may be so abnormal that their refusal to be hypnotized is a desperate resistance against the practitioner endeavouring to cure their neurotic symptoms.

That the hypnotic condition verges on a neurose is made evident by several of its characteristics.

The fact that it can be best induced in certain cases by a man of the Svengali type and that fakers have better percentages of success than scientific experimenters points to a childish regression and a father fixation. The mother fixation may explain satisfactorily the second method.

The regression is shown in many cases by the childhood memories which constitute the woof of the subject's talk unless the hypnotist imposes by suggestion a different topic.

All consciousness of time generally disappears in hypnosis and the abolition of time seems to cause the subject a great deal of satisfaction. This reminds us of the epileptic fits so well described by Dostoyevsky and in the côurse of which Mishkin, the Idiot, exulted in the thought that there would be no more time limitations

The majority of hypnotized subjects have a feeling of pressure all over their body which is a source of most pleasurable feelings.

The Freudians have come to the plausible conclusion that this is a memory from the prenatal days when the fetus was submitted in the mother's womb to an even pressure of similar character.

Many more points of similarity between neurotic and hypnotic states could be mentioned. Every neurose is a form of auto-suggestion. The subject imagines he has a large amount of evidence for certain obsessive thoughts and beliefs. At the end of an analysis, the evidence has been disintegrated and destroyed. The hypnotized subject who carries out some command given by the hypnotist will, if questioned, present excellent and plausible reasons for performing actions he cannot help performing. After being assisted in remembering the beginnings of the hypnotic scene, however, he will gradually regain his consciousness of all that transpired and realize that his "reasons" were an unconscious fabrication.

Just as a neurose creates physical symptoms through auto-suggestion, Charcot and the Nancy hypnotists have shown that almost any hysterical symptom can be induced under hypnose and a com-

[274]

parison of the two processes is extremely illuminating.

In acute neurotic cases there is even a form of refusal to be analysed which can be compared to the refusal to be hypnotized.

It happens sometimes, in the course of an analysis, that when the examination reaches a crucial point, the subject develops a physical ailment which for the time being or for a more or less extended period of time places him beyond the analyst's reach.

A subject may feel suddenly distressed and ask for permission to leave the room, or the appointments are postponed on account of some gastric or abdominal disturbance unconsciously improvised for the occasion.

Shall we then attempt to relieve neurotic symptoms through a procedure which affects so many neurotic traits?

The neurotic who consults a hypnotist is, after all, seeking a quick escape from reality, from effort, from responsibilities.

He sees in the practitioner treating him the parent image and "runs back to father or mother" regressing to the age at which he had all his problems solved and the responsibility never weighed very heavily on his shoulders. He seeks the line of

[275]

least effort. Too often an analyst has the impression brought to bear forcibly on him that the subject places himself in his hands and will hold him responsible henceforth for all the acts of his life.

Unable to lean upon his parents any longer the neurotic seeks a substitute for them.

Physician and analyst must see at once through the threadbare schemes of the subject and not encourage that attitude. They must bend all their energies to one end, to making the patient entirely independent from them.

Take one subject who feels weak and easily tired and hence unable to perform certain necessary and unpleasant tasks.

The hypnotist will repeat to him during each "trance" that he is strong, strong enough to do his work.

But the weak patient is weakened by complexes which hypnosis does not remove. Hence the probability is that after that form of treatment the patient, unable to really feel strong, because he is not strong, will adopt one of the negative attitudes I have described in a previous chapter, "I will act as though I were strong," after which he will engage, according to his temperament, in boasting or disparaging, bullying or scheming, to prove his inexistent strength to himself and others. He may

[276]

enter a slightly agitated maniac state, followed by the inevitable reaction, depression.

Many serious experimenters have come to the conclusion that we cannot suggest anything to a subject unless he unconsciously craves to do that very thing. Suggestions of unpleasant actions are either rejected or very ephemeral. Suggesting murder or suicide proves effective mainly in the movies. Lombroso saw his subjects wake up every time he ordered them to perform humiliating tasks or to assume degrading rôles.

Our ethical and social notions, our prejudices and fears dominate the hypnotic state as they do the waking state.

Not only is the hypnotic method dangerous for it encourages forms of regression which are the basis of the neuroses, but it is an inefficient and haphazard procedure.

How can we know what suggestion will be acceptable to the subject because unconsciously he has already accustomed himself to it and is expecting it? Must we make hundreds of experiments, each of which weakens the patient's will a little more, in order to strike by mere chance a suggestion which will be both beneficial and acceptable, hence durable?

This applies not only to the form of hypnotism

which implies suggestions from hypnotist to subject but to the hypnotic rest cure devised by Wetterstrand of Upsal. Wetterstrand simply put his patients asleep and kept them in that condition, sometimes for days and weeks, in a house especially
fitted for that purpose.

Sleepless subjects must have derived some comfort from that treatment, granted, however, that they
were not, in the course of that hypnotic sleep, tortured and weakened by anxiety dreams, one thing
which could not be prevented or checked. To the
average neurotic, on the other hand, that protracted
drowsiness must have offered a dangerous means of
escape from the reality which they should have been
trained to face.

In the course of an analysis, the analyst, as I said
before, is most careful not to offer any suggestions,
for suggestions would be accepted by friendly subjects in order to please the analyst, and by hostile
subjects to get rid of the analyst.

When asking the subject for his reactions to the
various stimulus words used for that purpose, the
analyst simply asks the impersonal question: what
comes to your mind when you hear this word?

He avoids forms of examination which would
practically dictate the proper answer to the patient,
such as: Does not this remind you of . . . ?

[278]

He listens carefully, patiently, uncritically though sympathetically.

He may have certain theories as to the subject's trouble, its cause, origin, character, etc., but he never airs them before the subject.

It may be objected that a certain amount of involuntary suggestion is quite unavoidable. The element designed unscientifically as personal magnetism plays in all human relations a part which cannot be minimized.

A letter to a daily paper which publishes health advice by a very bald physician revealed in an amusing way the illogical effects of personal impressions. The correspondent was anxious to find a tonic for his rapidly thinning hair, but wished to have his inquiry referred to another physician than Dr. X, for the latter's denuded skull made him in his estimation unfit to prescribe for his trouble.

As a matter of fact, a man affected by calvities is more likely to have investigated hair restorers than a man with a healthy shock of hair, but the person who wrote the letter I mentioned felt that in such matters he could not trust a bald physician.

An athletic physical instructor will easily impress his pupils with the probable excellence of his method and an analyst who seems unlikely to ever

[279]

be affected by any nervous ailments will create in his subject's mind a confidence which facilitates his work.

Jung says very frankly somewhere that practitioners who manage to invest themselves with the halo of the medicine man are wise in every respect. Not only do they have a large practice but they also obtain the best results. Dealing with neurotics, the medical exorcist shows to his subjects his full valuation of the "psychic" element when he gives them an opportunity to fasten their faith to his mysterious personality.

That type of healer generally has a large practice but I disagree with Jung as to the final, not the temporary, results of such cures.

Emotional cures have been observed in thousands of cases, but they are seldom lasting, for they eliminate the symptoms, not the deeper factors causing the symptoms to appear.

Powdering up a red nose will have strikingly good temporary effects but the only way to deal with that sympton is to cure the gastric disturbance which is responsible for it.

Analysis does not powder up red noses. It seeks to determine the line of least resistance for the development of a harmonious personality. It tries to find out what the neurotic's unconscious is striv-

[280]

ing for and actually doing in an abnormal way. After destroying the absurd reasons which the neurotic advances for his abnormal behaviour, it tries to determine in collaboration with the subject himself a positive, vital, socially beneficial guiding line.

But it does not begin to seek that guiding line until the subject has been made entirely free from his complexes.

And here again we must establish a sharp distinction between psychoanalysis and the talking cures made popular, especially in Europe, by the late Dr. Dubois, and which is little more than an attempt at suggestion in the waking state.

Dubois' system of therapy, which consists in giving to the subject moral reasons for his recovery and in discussing rationally his case, is temporarily efficient if the subject is deeply impressed with the practitioner's personality and is ready to yield to his arguments.

The Dubois method bans all conversation about the past and tries on every occasion to turn the subject's glance toward the future, which psychologically is correct, for the neurosis is a regression to the past and to outworn solutions.

That procedure is really the second part of the psychoanalytic treatment. But the first part of it cannot be skipped. Before erecting a building one must clear the ground of all obstructions and blast the rocks which stand in the way.

Conscious advice is very weak against the positive orders which come from our unconscious, and here again, as in the case of hypnotic commands, only that sort of advice for which the unconscious is prepared will find ready acceptance and be permanently followed.

Complex after complex must be disintegrated and the subject must first be made conscious that most of his unconscious cravings are not representative of the intellectual, social and ethical level on which he should stand but survivals of, or regressions to, conditions obtaining at lower, that is, more archaic levels.

Some of his unconscious cravings will be found to lead him along a straight, positive, path. His dreams prove especially valuable in determining what his aptitudes are as well as his abnormal modes of wishfulfilment.

The task of the analyst, after he has freed the subject from his thraldom to an archaic unconscious, is to select in an unprejudiced way from all the unconscious material brought to the surface that which is positive, which shows beneficial adaptability to the subject's environment, which is capable of gratifying in a socially useful way the various urges struggling for expression.

Both in the clearing of the ground and in the building of the new structure, the analyst proceeds scientifically, according to convincing evidential data.

Both reactions and dreams show him what the subject can actually do and is predisposed to do, what actual help and hindrance the subject may derive from his unconscious; dreams, in particular, registering minutely as they do, the subject's progress in regaining his freedom, reveal accurately the time when advice touching a positive guiding line can be given openly.

If you have to deal for instance with a subject in whom the egotistical trend is strongly marked, you must at first disintegrate the false growths whereby his craving expresses itself indirectly and abnormally. After which, when the subject has acquired full insight into his conduct and is re-shaping his attitudes accordingly, the analyst can encourage certain forms of activity offering positive gratification to the subject's egotism and yet fitting perfectly in the environment in which he must live.

A neurotic with a decided talent in some direction can be led from a negative life of disparagement, slander, bitterness, in which he is only re-

[283]

ducing others to a lower level, to a positive life of accomplishment, in which a development of his abilities will gain him fame and power.

In other words, hypnotism only offers to sufferers a negative escape from reality, psychoanalysis a permanent formula for exchanging a negative life for a positive one; hypnotism makes sufferers dependent upon the hypnotist, psychoanalysis makes them independent from the analyst.

And yet, there may be exceptional cases in which hypnotism may be used legitimately. While no physician believes in administering strong narcotics, no physician will hesitate to inject large doses of morphine into an unfortunate person who is, let us say, being crushed to death under a railroad train and cannot be lifted from under the wheels until emergency apparatus has come.

In a case, for instance, when a neurotic is incapacitated by some of his symptoms, such as a sick headache, from performing some important task upon which his livelihood or reputation depends, an analyst would have a sufficient excuse for saving his subject from the added strain which might be caused by failure. But that form of treatment should only be resorted to in a grave emergency with the understanding that the procedure shall not be repeated. For the majority of

[284]

neurotics would rather sleep than talk and would rather regress to their abnormal ideas than to submit them to the destructive fire of psychoanalytic conversation.

BIBLIOGRAPHY

The most authoritative book on the subject is Smith Ely Jelliffe's "The Technique of Psychoanalysis" (Nervous and Mental Disease Pub. Co.), a volume of 160 pages covering the following points: Material to be analysed; whom to analyse; the literature, sources and history of psychoanalysis; the analytic procedure; the Oedipus complex as a psychological measuring unit; the transference; the resistances; the overcoming of the conflicts; the socialization of the personality; the practical use of the patients' dreams in analysis, etc.

Poul Bjerre's "The Theory and Practice of Psychoanalysis" contains many practical suggestions and illustrations of the analytical procedure.

VII. THE FOUR SCHOOLS OF PSYCHOANALYSIS

CHAPTER 1: FREUD. THE PIONEER

There are few orthodox Freudians at the present day. Few analysts accept all the conclusions which the creator of psychoanalysis reached, but all of them without any exception accept his premises. There is a *psychoanalytic point of view* which is common to the four principal exponents of the science, Freud, Jung, Adler and Kempf.

I have told elsewhere how Freud gradually came to that point of view, discarding many of his earlier theories as new evidence compelled this most conscious and modest of scientists to revise his own findings.

This chapter will be devoted to a brief exposition of the Freudian theories. In the chapters devoted to Jung, Adler and Kempf, I shall endeavour to bring out further details of it by showing to what extent these scientists disagree with the great pioneer.

The Freudian point of view is presented principally in three of Freud's books, the "Three Contributions to the Sexual Theory," the "Psychopathology of Every Day Life" and the "Interpretation of Dreams." The lectures he delivered at Clark University when he visited the United States and his "Introduction to Psychoanalysis" supply laymen with a clear and intelligible summary of his theories.

Freud considers that a study of dreams is the surest way to penetrate man's unconscious. The dreams of children are very easily understood: they are invariably the fulfilment of wishes which were aroused in children during the day and were not satisfied. The dreams of adults present more difficulties. They undergo a process of distortion, of disguise. The idea which underlies them was meant for a quite different verbal expression.

The manifest dream content is a disguised substitute for the unconscious dream thoughts, and this disguise is the work of the defensive forces of the ego, of the resistances.

These prevent the repressed wishes from entering the consciousness in our waking hours, and even in the relaxation of sleep, they are still strong enough to force them to hide themselves under a mask, to don a symbolical disguise.

By studying the irruptive ideas which arise through free association, we can discover the actual dream thoughts.

They are no longer incomprehensible; they are

[290]

associated with the impressions of the day preceding the dream and appear as the fulfilment of ungratified wishes.

The manifest dream which we remember after waking may then be described as the *disguised* fulfilment of *repressed* wishes.

The analysis of dreams reveals, according to Freud, the unsuspected importance which impressions and experiences from early childhood exert on human beings. In the dream life of the adult, the child continues to live and retain all the traits and wishes he ever had, even those which he was obliged to abandon in later years. Dream study enables one to realize through what complicated processes of development, repression, sublimation and reaction the normal adult has gradually grown out of the child.

Anxiety dreams do not invalidate the theory of wish fulfilment, for anxiety is one of the ways in which the ego relieves itself of repressed wishes which have become too strong and, therefore, anxiety can easily be experienced if the dream has gone too far toward the fulfilment of an objectionable wish.

Faulty actions are another class of phenomena which throw much light upon the workings of our unconscious. The forgetting of things which one is supposed to know, like proper names, in certain cases, slips of the tongue, mistakes in writing or reading, the automatic execution of purposive acts in wrong situations, the loss or breaking of certain objects, all these are trifles for which no one before Freud had sought a psychological explanation and which had always been considered as the consequences of absent-mindedness, inattention, etc.

This should also include actions and gestures which the subject performs unknowingly, such as playing with objects (buttons, pencils), humming melodies, handling one's person or clothing and the like.

These insignificant actions are not without meaning. They spring from the same sort of repressed wishes which are at the bottom of our dreams.

Such investigation, Freud states, trace back the symptoms of mental disease with surprising regularity to impressions from the sexual life. They show that the pathogenic wishes are erotic cravings and that disturbances of the erotic sphere are the most important factors of mental disease.

Psychoanalysis may at first trace the symptoms, not to sexual happenings but to banal traumatic experiences. This distinction, however, loses its significance through other circumstances. The

[292]

analytic research work which is necessary for the thorough explanation and the complete cure of mental disease does not stop in any case with the experiences which coincided with the onset of the disease. It goes back in every case to the adolescence and childhood of the patient. Here only does Freud find the impressions and experiences which determine the later sickness. It is the incompatible, repressed wishes of childhood which lend their power to the creation of symptoms.

These mighty wishes of childhood are very generally sexual in their nature.

Sexual impulses do not enter the child's life at puberty; the child brings them with him into the world and from these, what we call the "normal" sexuality of the adult gradually develops.

The sexual impulse of the child is very complex and can be analysed into many components arising from different sources. It is not at first related to the function of reproduction. It enables the child to secure various forms of pleasurable sensations such as the auto-excitation of certain particularly sensitive parts of the body, genitals, rectum, skin and other surfaces. Thumb sucking is a good example of this form of gratification.

As in this first phase of the child's sexual life the child finds the gratification he seeks in his own body, Freud calls this period the period of auto-erotism.

Besides auto-erotic manifestations, Freud finds in the early life of the child impulse components of the *libido* which presuppose a second person as their object.

These impulses appear in opposed pairs, active and passive. The most important pairs of this group are sadism and masochism, the pleasure of inflicting pain and the pleasure of suffering pain, and the active and passive forms of exhibitionism.

From the passive form of exhibitionism is derived the impulse toward artistic or histrionic representation. From the active form, scientific curiosity.

The differences between the sexes play no very important part in the child's life and there is in every child a homosexual tendency.

The sexual life of the child, varied but inorganized, in which each single craving goes about seeking its satisfaction independently from the others, becomes gradually organized in two directions and, at the time of puberty, the definite sex of the individual is clearly determined.

The various cravings submit themselves to the primacy of the genital zone and the entire sexual life is taken over into the service of procreation.

[294]

Object choice prevails over auto-erotism and the love object satisfies all the separate cravings of the sex urge.

But many of the original components of that urge are given no share in the final shaping of the sexual life. Even before the advent of puberty, certain cravings had been submitted to the strongest repression by education. Shame, disgust, morality prevent the repressed cravings from asserting themselves.

Every process of development brings with itself the germ of pathological predispositions whenever it is inhibited, delayed or incompletely carried out. This is true of the sexual development. In some individuals it may not be completed and it may leave in its wake abnormalities or a predisposition to later diseases by the way of *regression.* Some cravings which have not fallen under the domination of the genital zone may cause a perversion. The original equality of the sexes may be maintained and homosexualism is the result.

The neuroses contain the same cravings found in perversions but in a negative form. Those cravings have undergone a repression but maintain themselves as complexes in the unconscious.

Exaggerated expression of a craving in very early life leads to a *fixation.*

[295]

The child takes both parents as an object of his erotic wishes but soon singles out one of them, following in that respect the example set by his parents, the father preferring his daughter, the mother, her son. The child reacts to that choice and if a son, wishes himself in the place of his father, if a daughter in the place of her mother.

The feelings aroused by such relations between parents and offspring are not only of a positive and affectionate nature but of a hostile and negative nature as well.

A situation ensues which can be roughly represented by the myth of Oedipus, who killed his father and married his mother.

This fixation which is submitted at an early age to a strong repression is to Freud's mind the central complex of every neurosis.

About the time when the child is still obsessed by this complex his attention is drawn towards the processes of reproduction and he begins to seek solutions for the question: where do children come from? Children build up at that time a number of pregnancy and birth theories which reappear in later life in many neuroses.

The neurotic disturbance is simply the individual's flight from a reality in which his repressed cravings cannot be gratified. The resist-

[296]

ance of the neurotic against any cure is due to the
fact that he is not certain that the substitute gratification offered him by his sickness can be replaced
in reality by something better.

The neurotic flight from reality takes place over
the path of regression, through a return to earlier
stages of life in which gratification was not lacking.
The regression is a twofold one, for the libido regresses not only to an earlier stage of development,
but also adopts primitive, archaic forms of expression.

We are all, whether we are normal or abnormal,
seeking an escape from reality. The strong, en-
ergetic man tries by dint of labour to make his
wishes come true and generally succeeds. If the
individual displeased with reality possesses artistic
talent he can transform his fancies into artistic
creations. The neurosis takes in our days the place
of the cloister in which the weak and disappointed
took refuge.

The neurosis has no psychic content of its own
which cannot be found in healthy minds. The
struggle for life leads either to success and health,
or to compensatory activities or to the neurosis.

Freud has divided mental disturbances into
neuroses, psychoneuroses and psychoses.

The true neuroses are anxiety neurosis and

neurasthenia. Their cause lies in the present and in the abnormal condition of the sexual function.

The psycho-neuroses are hysteria and the obsession neurosis, in which the real causative factors belong to the patients' early childhood.

In psychoneuroses as well as in neuroses the factors of the disturbance are sexual, but in the psychoneuroses the influence of heredity is more important.

Heredity finds its expression in a peculiar psychosexual constitution which asserts itself in an abnormally strong and many-sided instinctive life and a resultant sexual precocity.

Between the compelling instinct and the opposing force of sexual denial, the way is prepared for some disturbance which does not solve the conflict but seeks to escape it by changing the libidinous cravings into symptoms of disease.

Besides actual heredity, however, there is a pseudo-heredity which is after all the influence of the environment. Neurotic parents may not procreate neurotic children but they bring up their children to be neurotics.

Freud does not classify the psychoses according to their clinical picture but according to their mechanism, into *overpowering psychoses* and *defence psychoses*. In the former, the unconscious

[298]

has completely overcome the conscious and the ego has torn itself loose from some unbearable idea. For instance a girl disappointed in love imagined for two months that she was living with her lover and in that abnormal way had her wishes fulfilled.

The defence psychoses are characterized by the violent repression of an idea. In dementia praecox there is a withdrawal of the libido from the objects of the external world. Freud observed a group of paranoia cases arising from repression of painful memories. The libido fastening itself to the ego complex may lead to ideas of grandeur, which explains the connection between persecution mania and grandiose delusions. As far as the periodic melancholia is concerned, Freud asserts that it dissolves itself with unexpected frequency into obsessional ideas and obsessional affects.

In other words, insanity is no longer considered as a brain disease or as a set of absurd symptoms grouped in varying clinical pictures. Insanity is an abnormal asset for the insane, a dream from which he does not awaken and which supplies him with an abnormal form of wish-fulfilment.

The analytic treatment as outlined by Freud consists in letting the patient talk on any subject he pleases, since nothing can occur to him which does

not bear on the complex which the analyst is seeking. The patient often stops and pretends that he
has nothing more to say. This indicates that the
patient is holding back or rejecting certain ideas
because his unconscious resistance masquerades
as a critical judgment of the value of the ideas.
The patient can avoid that if he is warned in advance and told not to pass any judgment on the
ideas that come to his mind, however unessential,
irrelevant, nonsensical or personally unpleasant
they may be.

These irruptive ideas which the patient values
little, "are to the analyst like the ore which can be
transformed through simple processes into valuable metal." If one desires to gain in a short time
a preliminary knowledge of the patient's repressed
complexes, the examination can be conducted with
the help of association experiments.

This procedure is to the analyst what qualitative
analysis is to the chemist. It may be dispensed
with in the therapy of neurotic patients, but it is
indispensable in the study of the psychoses.

This is followed by dream study and the close
observation of the patient's involuntary, faulty actions, etc.

Freud attaches a great importance to the phenomenon known as the *transference* which he con-

siders as further evidence of the sexual forces which
are at the bottom of the neurosis.

The patient, he says, directs toward the person
of the physician a great amount of tender emotion,
often mixed with enmity, which has no foundation
in any real relation, and must be derived in every
respect from the old wish-fancies of the patient
which have become unconscious.

Every fragment of his emotional life, which can
no longer be called back into memory, is accordingly lived over by the patient in his relation to
the physician, and only by living it over in the
transference is he convinced of the power of those
unconscious sexual stimuli. The symptoms
which, to use a chemical expression, are the precipi-
tates of earlier love experiences, using the word
love in its broadest sense, can only be dissolved in
the high temperature of the experience of transference and transformed into other psychic products.

The phenomenon of transference is not created
by the psychoanalytic treatment. It arises spon-
taneously in all human relations and in the relations of the patient to the physician. It is every-
where the bearer of therapeutic influences and the
stronger it is the less one is aware of its presence.

Psychoanalysis does not create it but simply

[301]

reveals it to consciousness and avails itself of it to direct the psychic processes toward a certain goal.

People ignorant of the analytic technique often express the fear that by causing certain unconscious cravings to rise to consciousness those cravings may overpower the patient's ethical strivings and rob him of his cultural acquisitions.

Experience teaches, Freud states, that the physical and mental power of a wish whose repression has failed, is incomparably stronger when it remains unconscious than when it is made conscious. The unconscious wish cannot be influenced and is not hindered by strivings in the opposite direction, while the conscious wish is inhibited by other conscious wishes of an opposite nature.

What then becomes of the cravings which were set free by analysis? How can they be made harmless for the individual?

The craving is generally "consumed" during the analysis by the correct mental activity of opposite wishes which are conscious and more valuable socially. Repression is replaced by condemnation. This is easy, Freud thinks, as we have only in the majority of the cases, to efface the effects of earlier developmental stages of the ego.

Analysis may also reveal that some unconscious

cravings can be gratified in ways which would have been found earlier if the development of the individual had not been disturbed. The mere extirpation of infantile wishes is not the ideal aim of development, for the neurotic loses, through his repressions, many sources of mental energy which could have been utilized for his character building and his life activities.

Sublimation is a process which directs the energy of the infantile wish-stimuli toward a higher goal, eventually no longer sexual. The components of the sexual urge have a great capacity for sublimation and can exchange their sexual goal for one more remote and socially valuable. "To the utilization of the energy reclaimed in such a way, in the activities of our mental life, we probably owe the highest cultural achievements. As long as an impulse is repressed, it cannot be sublimated. After the removal of the repression, the way to sublimation is open."

BIBLIOGRAPHY

The following books by the founder of the psycho-analytic science must be read before one can acquire a clear understanding of Freud's doctrines:

FREUD, S.—"Three Contributions to the Theory of Sex" (Nervous and Mental Disease Pub. Co.)

Freud, S.—"The Interpretation of Dreams" (Macmillan).

Freud, S.—"The Psychopathology of Everyday Life" (Macmillan).

Freud, S.—"Wit and the Unconscious" (Moffat, Yard).

Freud, S.—"The Origin and Development of Psychoanalysis" (Clark University).

Freud, S.—"The History of the Psychoanalytic Movement" (Nervous and Mental Disease Pub. Co.).

Freud, S.—"Introduction to Psychoanalysis" (Boni and Liveright).

To understand the application of Freud's theories to purely morbid states one should consult Hitschmann's "Freud's Theories of the Neuroses" (Moffat, Yard), a most reliable book of reference.

CHAPTER II: JUNG. THE ZURICH SCHOOL

Dr. Carl G. Jung of Zurich, Switzerland, one of Freud's disciples, has developed his master's views, broadening them out in certain respects but imparting to them in other respects a great deal of vagueness.

Freud's conception of the libido does not satisfy Jung. He conceived that urge as a force reaching far beyond the confines of sexuality or love even in their broadest sense. To him this force is a mysterious thing, similar to Bergson's Vital Urge, and which manifests itself not merely through sex and other hedonist activities, but through organic growth and development, and through all mental and intellectual activities.

He agrees with Freud that the instinct of reproduction is at the basis of hundreds of manifestations which at the present day seem to have completely lost all the sexual significance they once had, but he refuses, on account of their present character, to designate them as sexual.

In place of a sexual viewpoint, Jung introduces into abnormal psychology an *energic* viewpoint.

The first manifestation of the libido or vital energy is the instinct of nutrition. From this stage the libido slowly develops through the many activities of the act of sucking into the sexual function. Hence he does not consider the act of sucking as a sexual act. The pleasure derived from sucking the mother's nipple cannot be considered as a sexual pleasure but as a nutritional pleasure, for Jung does not see anywhere any evidence that pleasure in itself is sexual.

It is because the libido attaches itself to an object or withdraws itself from it that the object interests us or appeals to us. The object itself is indifferent. The neurotic has no conscious reason for the outflow or the withdrawal of his libido, but when there is an exaggerated interest for one object, there is a consequent lack of energy elsewhere.

The second point on which Jung disagrees with Freud is the meaning of the childish manifestations of sexuality which Freud calls "polymorphous perverse" because of their similarity to the abnormal phenomena of adult life known as perversions.

Jung refuses to use the word perverse in connection with those infantile activities. They are to his mind the gradual enfoldment of sexuality. He divides life into three periods: the presexual period extending to the third or fourth year, in which the

[306]

libido is mainly occupied with nutrition and growth, and corresponds roughly to the caterpillar stage of the butterfly.

Then comes the prepubertal stage, from the fourth year to the age of puberty, followed by the period of maturity.

In the presexual stage, the "polymorphous perverse" activities arise from the general broadening of the libido which is no longer at the exclusive service of nutrition and begins to flow through many other channels. The childish habits are abandoned gradually, which means that a large amount of libido is withdrawn from them.

If on the other hand the libido in its extension from nutrition to sex is arrested or retarded, a fixation may result, creating a disharmony, for the physical growth of the child cannot wait and never stops. A discrepancy arises between the infantile character of the child's emotional life and the needs of the more mature individual and the seed is sown for some maladaptation of the neurotic type.

The child uses up a great amount of energy in day dreaming which compensates him for the thousand things which the world is denying him or rather taking away from him.

As the human being passes from childhood into adulthood, the increasing demands which life

[307]

makes upon him compel him to abandon the world of fancies in which he spent so many hours. There again there may be a lingering of the libido in the phantasy stage and this leads to a condition called introversion. The introvert is characterized by the fact that his libido is turned toward his own personality and that he regards everything from the point of view of his personality. The introvert lingers on situations and experiences which are a thing of the past, which are no longer of any import and which obscure to him the actual situation he should face.

This constitutes another form of maladaptation to practical life with its various social aspects.

The dominant factor in the child's life are the parents.

At this point, Jung again disagrees with Freud. Jung admits that there are many neurotic persons, who, in their infancy and childhood, showed unmistakable neurotic traits which in later life became more deeply marked. And he realizes also that the parents wield on the child's destiny, by their affection or lack of affection, wrong example, etc., an influence which is decisive for the child's future.

The child's mentality may be so moulded by early influences that in later life he will constantly seek in the actual world conditions which dominated in the family circle and will never be satisfied until he thinks he has drawn near that goal.

But the adult is not conscious of those influences and may actually consider himself absolutely free from such tyranny, the more so as he often realizes the profound outward difference between present and past conditions and fails to notice their essential similarity.

Therefore, Jung does not consider that the *actual* parents are the *actual* factors in a subject's attitude to life and its problems, but rather the distorted, often idealized, images of the parents, the *father imago* and the *mother imago*.

To Jung, the Oedipus Complex is a purely symbolic situation in which the mother has absolutely no sexual significance for the child.

It is not the mere existence of this complex, Jung writes, which characterizes the neurotic, for *everybody has it in his unconscious,* but the neurotic's strong attachment to it. This so-called fixation is probably a normal phenomenon. The fact that the neurotic seems markedly influenced by it shows that it is less a matter of fixation than of a peculiar ise which he makes of his infantile past. He exaggerates its importance and attributes to it a great artificial value.

The jealousy which even very young children

[309]

may show toward their father more or less corresponds to the displeasure which certain animals,
dogs, for example, show in regard to strangers ap-
proaching their masters or the caresses their masters
may lavish on other dogs, cats, etc.   Children probably appreciate their mother most as a source of
food, protection and physical comfort.   Later,
when eroticism begins to develop, the male child
tends to prefer the mother, the female child the
father, the male child experiencing something akin
to sexual jealousy toward his father, the female
child toward her mother.

As puberty is attained, male and female child
free themselves from their too exclusive attachment
for their parents and upon the extent of their detachment depends their future well being.

This disentanglement is often accompanied by a
severe struggle and a mental and physical crisis
which Jung designates as the stage of self-sacrifice.
In that period the childish tendencies and forms of
love are sacrificed in order that the energy they
consume may be freed and turned toward self-
fulfilment aims.

We now reach another important point whereon
Jung separates himself from Freud.

To Freud the many repressions which take place
before and during the stage characterized by Jung

as the stage of self-sacrifice result in the accumulation of unconscious material constantly seeking an outlet. Hence to Freud, dreams are in their essence a symbolic veil for repressed desires which are in conflict with the ideals of the personality.

To Jung the dream is a subliminal picture of the psychological condition of the individual in his waking state. It represents a résumé of the subliminal association material which is brought together by the momentary psychological situation. The volitional meaning of the dream which Freud calls the repressed desire is to Jung a means of expression.

The activity of the consciousness, speaking biologically, represents the psychological effort which the individual makes in adapting himself to the conditions of life. His consciousness endeavours to adjust itself to the necessities of the moment. In other words, there are tasks that the individual must perform, obstacles he must overcome. In many cases he is at a loss to find a solution and hence tends to refer to previous experiences of a more or less similar nature. We always try to understand the unknown which lies in the future in terms of the known which happened in the past.

As Jung sees no reasons for supposing that the unconscious follows laws different from those rul-

ing conscious thought, he believes that the unconscious arrives at an understanding of the unknown
by assimilating it to something which is known.
When America was first discovered by the
Spaniards, the Indians took the horses of the con-
querors for huge pigs, for they were familiar with
the appearance of pigs, had never seen horses and
hence drew comparisons between the unknown
horses and the well known pigs.

Hence the wealth of symbols used in dreams.

It is then the *present* conflict which, according
to Jung, dominates our dream states and supplies
their content.

And it is the *present* conflict, too, Jung thinks,
which causes the onset of the neurosis. Jung rejects the Freudian view according to which the infantile past is the direct causes of the neurosis.

Jung thinks that the regression to infantile or
childish forms of thought or action is prompted by
the patient's desire to withdraw as far as possible
from the present.

The conflict is produced by some important task
which is essential for the fulfilment of the individual's destiny and which the subject refuses to
perform.

A sensitive and somewhat inharmonious character will always meet with special difficulties and
[312]

with greater obstacles than a perfectly normal and more resistant individual. For the neurotic, there are no established ways, as his aims and tasks are apt to be of a highly individual character. He tries to follow the more uncontrolled half-conscious ways of normal people, not fully realizing his own critical nature which imposes upon him more effort than the normal person is required to exert. There are children who show their increased sensitiveness and inadaptability in the very first weeks of their life by their difficulty in taking the breast, by their exaggerated nervous reactions.

This predisposition is the cause of the first resist-ances against adaptation. In such cases the libido does not find its appropriate outlet and replaces modern and acceptable forms of adaptation by some abnormal, primitive forms.

Infantile fantasies determine the form and fur-ther development of a neurosis but they do not constitute the origin of the neurosis. The fact that the patient himself may consider infantile fancies as the cause of his neurosis does not prove that he is right in his belief or that a theory following the same belief is right either. The fact that infantile fancies are exaggerated and put into the foreground is simply a consequence of the stored-up energy or libido.

The psychological trouble in neurosis and neurosis itself can be considered as an act of adaptation that has failed. A neurosis is, from a certain point of view, an attempt at self-cure.

Jung's view of the neurosis does not prevent him from adhering to the Freudian mode of analysis. The analyst, according to Jung, must not imagine that, by unravelling the infantile fancies he is unearthing the end roots of the disease. But he must uproot those fancies because the energy which the patient needs for his health, that is, for his adaptation, is attached to them.

By means of psychoanalysis the connection between the conscious life and the libido in the unconscious is re-established. Thus this unconscious libido is placed anew at the service of conscious activity. Only in this way can split-off energy become again available for the accomplishment of the necessary tasks of life.

To Jung, psychoanalysis is no longer a mere reduction of the individual to his primitive sexual wishes but "a high moral task of immense educational value." It should not occupy itself with conflicts for which an external solution can be found unless it can adjust them through an internal solution. For example, some man dissatisfied with

[314]

his home life may think that all his difficulties would disappear if he married another woman. But the old Adam would probably bungle the new union as it bungled the old one. A real solution for many such conflicts only comes from within, and only then because the patient has been brought to a new standpoint.

For example, the conflict between love and duty must be solved upon that particular plane of character where love and duty are no longer in opposition. The familiar conflict between instinct and conventional morality must be solved in such a way that both factors are taken into account and this is only possible through a change of character.

Jung regards the question of the doctor's remaining true to his scientific convictions as rather unimportant in comparison with the question as to how he can best help his patient.

The analyst must be a teacher of ethics. Young neurotics must be made to realize that their search for a more valuable personality is often a cloak for the evasion of biological duty. Older patients looking back too obstinately toward the sexual valuation of youth may be simply retreating from a duty which demands the recognition of social values. In most cases the "canalization of the

[315]

libido" for the fulfilment of life's simple duties suffices to reduce to nothing many exaggerated desires.

At the same time, Jung calls our attention to the fact that the question is not as simple as that and cannot always be solved in terms of "morality." "Immoral" tendencies cannot always be removed by analysis. On the contrary, some of them appear often more clearly and hence one must come to the conclusion that they belong to the individual's biological duties. This is no longer a problem for pathologists but for sociologists. This is especially true of certain sexual claims. Nature does not content herself with theories. At the present day we have no real sexual morality, only a *legal* attitude toward sexuality. Just as the early Middle Ages had no business ethics but only certain prejudices and a legal standpoint.

This obscure feeling that a new, more progressive world is needed constitutes, at times, a part of the neurotic complication. We must not forget that the moral law of today will be cast tomorrow into the melting pot to the end that it may serve at some future time as the basis of some new ethical structure.

So it comes that there are many neurotics whose delicacy of feeling prevents them from being in

[316]

agreement with present-day morality and who cannot adapt themselves to civilization as long as their moral code has gaps, the filling of which is the crying need of the age.

Jung thinks that in many cases neurotics are neurotics, not because they are unsatisfied sexually or have not found the right mate or because they still are suffering from a fixation on their infantile sexuality: the real cause for their neurosis is, in many cases, their inability to recognize the work that is waiting for them, of helping to build up a new civilization.

In the past nothing can be altered, and in the present very little, but the future is ours. The neurotic is ill not because he has lost his old faith but because he has not as yet found a new form for his finest aspirations.

BIBLIOGRAPHY

Beginners will find Jung's theories presented in a very lucid way in Beatrice M. Hinckle's introduction to Jung's "Psychology of the Unconscious" (Moffat, Yard). For more detail, consult C. G. Jung's "Analytical Psychology" (Moffat, Yard) in which the Swiss analyst not only discusses his position in regard to the various problems of psychoanalysis but brings out the main points on which he disagrees with Freud and Adler. His correspondence with Dr. Loy, which is included in this volume, will prove most interesting, as it reveals to the reader the mental evolution which led Jung from the practice of hypnotism to that of psychoanalysis. C. J. Jung's "The Association Method" (Clark University) explains very clearly some of the methods of analytical examination. Advanced students will find the development of his thought and its applications to religion and folk lore in his "Psychology of the Unconscious" and in his "Studies in Word-Association" (Moffat, Yard).

CHAPTER III: ADLER. INDIVIDUAL PSYCHOLOGY

Adler does not call himself a psychoanalyst. After breaking away from the Freudian camp he designated his research work and his methods of psychiatry as Individual Psychology. The term has merits, for there are no cut-and-dried rules in the study and treatment of mental disturbances and every case must be approached from a different angle. It has not, however, been used by any one else in the literature of psychoanalysis.

Freud considers human life as the result of the play of unconscious forces which drive us blindly and which we are in no way capable of leading or regulating. The repressed desires which are constantly seeking an outlet and which by creating an abnormal outlet for themselves upset at times our mental balance, serve no definite purpose.

Jung, dissatisfied with this form of psychological fatalism, contended that the neurosis was an unsuccessful attempt at adjusting one's conduct to the problems of the present.

Adler thinks that all the forces of the individual

[319]

are tending toward a definite goal and that in every manifestation of life we can find traces of a dominating or guiding idea.

In other words, Freud emphasized the importance of the past, Jung that of the present, Adler that of the future.

To Adler the most minute trait of psychic life is permeated with a purpose-force. Every psychic event bears the impress, or in other words is a symbol of a uniformly directed plan of life which only comes to light more clearly in the neurosis. But none of the neurotic traits are characteristic of the neurotic exclusively. The neurotic shows no single idiosyncrasy which cannot be proved to exist in the healthy individual, although it may only be revealed to the subject of the analyst through analysis.

Adler reached his psychological viewpoint after studying the effect which some organic inferiority has on the mental and physical health of the individual. While Freud started in life as a hypnotist and under the influence of Charcot and Bernheim, Adler's first work was a monograph on Organ Inferiority.

Nature is constantly at work to compensate for all the deficiencies found in the organism. If one kidney is removed the other grows larger and does as much work as two did. If some of the heart valves are destroyed the muscular activity of the heart increases and thus the blood stream is kept in motion at the proper rate. But nature does more than that. An organ's capacity for work depends not only upon its physical condition but on the nerve impulses sent to it by the central nervous system. A defective organ may be made to function properly through a vigorous exercise of the will. The weakened organ is likely to become, on that account, unduly sensitive and in this peculiarity we can find the roots of nervous suffering.

A patient suffering from nervous gastric or intestinal trouble, for instance, is often one who once suffered from such a disturbance and was cured. The ailment may have affected him in his early childhood, but the memory of it has been retained unconsciously and is recalled when the occasion arises.

The neurotic, Adler says, suffers from a feeling of incompleteness for which he seeks compensation. The entire picture of the neurosis and all its symptoms are influenced if not provoked by an imaginary fictitious goal. It is not the "libido" which is the motive force behind the phenomena of the neurosis, but the wish to be a complete man. The libido, the sex cravings and the tendencies to perversions become subjugated by this power. Adler in this respect agrees with Nietzsche's theory of the will-to-power and will-to-seem and also with some of the older writers who held that the feeling of pleasure originates in a sense of power and the feeling of pain in a sense of weakness.

Adler objects to Freud's contention that the neurosis has a sexual origin. The sexual picture, he says, deceives easily the normal person and more easily yet the neurotic, but it must not deceive the psychologist. The neurotic phenomenon is given a sexual tinge by the antithesis "masculine-feminine" which has gradually imposed itself upon human thinking and which obsesses neurotic thinking. The assumption (now less generally spread, but universal before the feminist movement began to check it), that masculine meant also superior and strong, and that feminine meant inferior and weak, is gospel truth to the neurotic and a source of great suffering.

The sexual trend in the neurotic's fancies and in his life leads toward the masculine goal. The whole picture of the sexual neurosis is simply a graphic presentation of the distance separating the patient from the imaginary masculine goal which he is trying to reach.

The neurotic is not, as Freud thought, obsessed

[322]

by infantile wishes which come to life nightly through his dreams. For those infantile wishes are themselves subordinated to the fictitious goal, and adapt themselves to symbolic expression for the sake of convenience.

A sickly girl who, during her childhood, was conscious of her insecurity and who has to rely entirely on her father as far as her present and future security is concerned, tends to usurp some of her mother's privileges and may imagine the entire situation in the form of an incest; she is taking the place of her mother in her father's affections; she is almost as important to her father as though she were her father's wife. She may never marry, for marriage with a stranger would not mean the security she finds with her father, who is stronger, wiser, and makes no physical demands likely to humiliate her ego. With a little imagination she may easily conjure up the symbolic picture of an incestuous relation.

Freud saw in this fantasy a re-birth of infantile wishes. Adler sees in this attempt to reach into the remote past, in that tendency of the neurotic to abstraction and symbolization, a clever unconscious scheme to attain security, to vouchsafe to the ego the greatest amount of gratification and to reach the masculine goal.

How do neurotic symptoms originate? Why does the patient wish to be a man and constantly seek to prove to himself his virility? Why does he need so many egotistical forms of gratification?

Because, Adler answers, there stands at the threshold of the neurosis a threatening feeling of inferiority and life becomes unbearable unless the neurotic can look forward to a situation which assures him, normally or abnormally, safety and superiority.

The neurotic individual, aside from his purely neurotic symptoms, will easily become conspicuous owing to his evident inability to adapt himself to his environment. The consciousness of his weak point obsesses him to such a degree that often without knowing it, he begins to build over it a protective structure.

His sensitiveness becomes more acute; he learns to discern relationships which escape others, he exaggerates his cautiousness, anticipates all sorts of unpleasant consequences when he starts out to do something or suffers some injury; he endeavours to hear and to see more than others can hear or see; he belittles himself; he becomes insatiable, economical, constantly strives to extend the boundaries of his influence and power over space and time and

[324]

soon loses the peace of mind and the freedom from prejudice which guarantee mental health.

His distrust of himself and others, his envy and maliciousness become more and more pronounced. He either tries to gain the upper hand in cruel, aggressive ways or he endeavours to dominate his environment by his very humility and submissiveness.

Freud points out that the neurosis is a means of escape from reality. Adler stresses the fact that to the neurotic, life is nothing but a dangerous adventure. Not only must he escape that danger but he must construct a strong system of defence that will protect him against it. The man for whom every woman constitutes a temptation may develop in his mind an obsessive fear of syphilis, after which he thinks himself secure behind that protective wall; the unhappily mated wife escapes intercourse which is odious to her by developing vague pains in her sexual organs; an overworked country preacher runs away and becomes for a period of ime a fruit seller; the bed-ridden neurotic who finds life too monotonous has peculiar attacks, rushes to a window, threatens to commit suicide and hence secures the constant company of a nurse.

All these neurotic symptoms are ready-for-use attitudes. The patient is not shamming. He unconsciously remembers earlier defects, earlier sieges of sickness and reproduces them when an emergency arises. He unconsciously produces the required symptom as the fingers of a pianist reproduce without any conscious effort a certain combination of notes which has been carefully memorized.

Adler foresees the objections which such a theory is bound to bring forth. How can trigeminal neuralgia, insomnia, paralysis, sick headaches, etc., afford the neurotic any form of gratification? Because neurotic symptoms are in the majority of cases sure means for obtaining mastery over another person. And to that craving for power and superiority the neurotic is as ready to sacrifice his comfort as normal human beings are to undergo hardships in order to attain some of their ideals. The neurotic's absurd goal is an abnormal ideal, but to him an ideal just the same.

To Adler, dreams only acquire a meaning when we consider them as a symbol of life. The dream is a sketchlike reflection of psychic attitudes and reveals to the investigator the manner in which the dreamer regards certain problems.

The dream is not the fulfilment of some infantile wishes, but a neurotic way of securing for the ego an easy form of gratification, and of solving prob-
[326]

lems which to the neurotic appear too complicated. Repeated dreams of the same type reveal the course followed by the fictitious guiding line. They indicate various attempts at solving one problem and hence betray a characteristic feeling of uncertainty.

The analysis of dreams appears as essential to Adler as to Freud as a part of the analytic treatment. Adler, however, rejects entirely the literal Freudian interpretation and shares some of Jung's symbolistic views.

The incest motive he thinks is as little real in dreams as it is in the waking life of the individual. When man dreams for instance of intercourse with his mother, he is just running back to her for protection as he did when a child. The fact that near relations appear so often in our dreams in sexual situations is due to the very make up of our unconscious.

There are in our unconscious several layers of memory pictures and the deeper we go, the fewer pictures we find, until arriving at the bottom we only find the parents, the first pictures the individual ever beheld. That those are more likely to recur than any others and to be used symbolically whenever our archaic, primitive unconscious needs human types to symbolize men or women, is easily understood.

While Freud stressed the love motive, Adler stresses the power motive and thus explains the neurotic's strange inability to love, his strange tendency to become self-centred.

Intent on protecting himself against all the perils of life, the neurotic is constantly on his guard. To surrender to any tender feeling would mean to him to submit to some other ego.

Love to him is only another danger to be warded off, a weak spot in his defence system through which the enemy, life, might enter to defeat him. The neurotic will either try to be an ascetic or a Don Juan. As a mysogynist he will proclaim his superiority over every woman, as a Don Juan he will proclaim woman's frailty and his irresistible virility. In either direction he will be found totally lacking in measure.

Artistic creation, to Adler, is simply another form of compensation for the individual's organic shortcomings. Organs of slight inferiority may develop, he says, greater functional capacities than normal organs.

All mental operations have a tendency to concentrate on the weak organ in order to protect it from harm. Singers, speakers, actors, he says, have generally recovered from some organic defect which in their infancy and childhood prompted

[328]

them to exercise their defective throat, tongue or lips. Musicians may have been overexercising a defective ear. Painters became interested in colours and nuances owing to their originally weak eyes. Adler calls our attention to the fact that Demosthenes, who became Greece's greatest orator, struggled for many years with an impediment in his speech, that Mozart and Beethoven suffered from severe ear trouble, that Bruckner's ears were stigmatized by moles, and that there are more cases of defective vision among pupils of art schools than among any other classes of the population.

He even holds that our sense of inferiority determines the profession we embrace in real life and mentions that many excellent chefs he examined were suffering or had recovered from acute gastric trouble. Their inferiority caused them to pay special attention to food and its preparation, etc.

The social bearing of Adler's doctrines is briefly indicated in the preface to the second edition of his Neurotic Constitution: "Our Individual Psychology has gone far beyond the dead line of descriptive psychology; to understand a man means to save him from the errors into which he is led by his sore, frantic but futile craving to be like unto God and to make him amenable to the unshakable logic of human community life, to instil into him the community sense."

BIBLIOGRAPHY

The best résumé of Adler's theories will be found in Poul Bjerre's "Theory and Practice of Psychoanalysis." The only works of Adler's which are accessible to English readers are his monograph on "Organ Inferiority and its Psychic Compensation" (Nervous and Mental Disease Pub. Co.) which contains many case histories upon which he was to build his later theories. His "Neurotic Constitution" (Moffat, Yard) is less a book than a series of studies of the neurotic life from several points of view.

CHAPTER IV: KEMPF. DYNAMIC MECHANISM

Valuable as their theories are, one cannot help feeling that Freud's and Jung's mode of thinking is still closely related to that of the academic psychologists. They give the impression that the mental and the physical are two separate entities. The term *conversion* used by Freud to designate the physical symptoms accompanying certain emotions seems to imply a duality in organic manifestations which, to modern scientists, appears totally unfounded.

When Freud and Jung speak of *libido, cravings, censor,* etc., they are almost as vague and unconvincing as Bergson when he speaks of the *vital urge.*

Adler felt the necessity of establishing a more intimate connection between physical and mental manifestations, but he did not make the mechanism of *compensation* clearer to his readers than Freud did the mechanism of *conversion.*

It will be only when we know what part of

the organism "produces" an emotion and, reciprocally, what part of the organism is affected by a given emotion, that we shall visualize clearly the relations between "mind" and "body." Then we shall understand the meaning of the *vital urge* and of the *libido;* then, the so-called "nervous" disturbances as well as consciousness and its content (thought) shall lose their mystery.

Edward J. Kempf, of Saint Elizabeth Hospital, Washington, D. C., attacks the problem from a new and original point of view.

Kempf states frankly his dislike of the term *libido.* Although that term attempts to represent graphically the energic constitution of man and his love of life, it lacks clearness, for the human mind cannot very well conceive of a *process* as such, unless there is some *thing* that *proceeds.*

The concept of electricity would be hazy indeed, were it not that we can visualize dynamos, wires, sparks, bulbs and many other visible, tangible, etc., means of production or manifestation of the force called electricity.

In order to explain the great physiological changes which influence human thought and behaviour and the biological nature of man, Kempf has developed a conception of the personality based on the reflex actions of the autonomic nervous system.

To him the human organism is a biological machine which assimilates, conserves, transforms and expends energy. All those operations are regulated by the autonomic apparatus which keeps in touch with the environment through the projicient sensori-motor nervous system.

As the autonomic apparatus becomes conditioned (trained) to have acquisitive and avertive tendencies toward its environment, according to which cravings are active in a given situation, the organism's behaviour is the resultant of a compromise between the opposed cravings.

The importance of the brain is greatly minimized by this conception. Experiments have proved that the same form of behaviour is not always due to the activity of the same brain cells and the theories which localize in certain regions of the brain the controlling forces of all human conduct must be abandoned.

According to Kempf, brain and personality, so long associated in popular parlance, must no longer be considered as interchangeable terms. In fact, every part of the body contributes something to the personality and to its consciousness of itself.

Should some one lose a limb or a group of

[333]

muscles, he would lose at the same time an important part of his personality. This would manifest itself in the manner in which he would adjust himself to the stresses of daily life, what he would try to do and feel compelled to avoid, etc.

Analysis alone would reveal that fact; the natural readjustment of the remaining muscles would prevent any gross change from being observable.

For instance, the loss of the eyes and arms would greatly reduce the ability to understand new machinery, new situations and probably reduce to an enormous extent the power of recalling experiences in which the eyes and hands played a predominant part, such as writing, etc.

Because most of our thoughts are dependent upon our muscle sense, it may be said that we actually think with our muscles. If we allow ourselves to become aware of the visual image of an automobile, we are aware that it is moving, because the muscles of the eyeball shift the image by modifying their postural tensions.

Sometimes the muscles of the neck may contribute more information by moving the head.

If we are pushing the automobile ourselves, the muscles of the body come into play to furnish other images and if we are pushing it along a cold, wet, muddy road, the sensations of cold, wetness and mud arise from the tactile receptors of our legs.

But such a perfect correlation between our autonomic apparatus and the sensori-motor system is a gradual acquisition of the human being in the course of it development.

At birth, we have a well-developed, well-balanced, autonomic apparatus and a poorly coordinated sensori-motor system. The autonomic apparatus, however, begins immediately to coordinate and control the sensori-motor system in order to master its environment.

A most important factor begins to exert pressure upon the infant from the very minute of its birth and exerts it throughout life. It is the incessant pressure of the social herd, which modifies the autonomic apparatus and compels it to adopt less and less primitive, more and more civilized and indirect methods of satisfying the various human cravings.

The tone or tension produced by the autonomic apparatus in the muscles which move our body and limbs determines largely the content of our consciousness or thoughts.

This leads us to a complete reversal of the view held by the academic philosophers and psychological laboratory observers.

According to them the emotions are one of the results of the mind's contemplation of phenomena taking place within or without the organism. "Bodily" reactions and "mental" reactions take place *after* the emotion has been experienced.

James and Lange advanced the theory that our feeling of bodily changes, following the perception of a stimulus, *is* the emotion. Kempf goes further and states that if we experience an emotion, it is because some parts of the autonomic apparatus have assumed a certain tension which produces the emotion. As evidence, he cites the fact that we are at times awakened at night by fearful tensions whose cause is unknown and then awaken to find that there is some one in our room. Nursing mothers experience vigorous disturbances in their sleep long before they become aware that their child is in distress. We become conscious of images of urinating in our dreams and find upon awakening, that uncomfortable tensions of the bladder have been active for some time owing to the accumulation of urine.

Kempf's theory of the dynamic mechanism is worded as follows:

"Whenever any segment of the autonomic-affective apparatus is forced into a state of hypertension through the necessities of metabolism or endogenous or exogenous stimuli, the hypertense seg-

[336]

ment gives off a stream of emotion or affective crav-ing which compels the projicient apparatus to so adjust the exteroceptors in the environment as to acquire stimuli which have the capacity to produce comfortable postural readjustments in those au-tonomic segments."

In other words, whenever autonomic nerves, for instance, the nerves causing the contractions of the stomach known as hunger, are made extremely tense by the sight or smell of food, they produce a strong emotion or desire which compels the sensori-motor nerves to apply the mouth to food, after which the tension of the autonomic nerves is relieved.

Kempf maintains that this biologic principle or law is the foundation of all human and animal be-haviour, to be seen throughout all its workings, whether brief and trivial or prolonged and elabor-ate. "The seeking and creating follows the co-rollary 'to obtain a maximum of autonomic grati-fication with a minimum expenditure of energy,' thus developing increasing skill and power, exten-sion of influence and assurance of comfort and an increasing margin of safety from liability to failure."

Most of the nervous tensions originating in the autonomic apparatus have as their biological aim the acquisition of appropriate pleasant stimulations and the avoidance of destructive unpleasant ones; for instance, they direct us toward food and away from some danger. They are relieved only when their objective stimulus is attained.

In certain cases the object is unattainable, being socially tobooed or having passed beyond our reach, as for example when a loved person dies. In such cases, tensions will remain unrelieved and become seriously distressing as well as dangerous for our mental and physical health. Among other things, they disturb the blood supply to certain organs and hence weaken them in their struggle against the bacteria of infectious diseases.

In case of tuberculosis, pneumonia, typhoid, excessive fatigue, an exaggerated emotional tension may be fatal. In other words, the individual who represses certain cravings because they are ungratifiable or for fear of the influence their gratification may have on his social standing, tends to have organs which are more liable to disease.

The struggle between conflicting cravings was considered by psychologists of the old school as taking place in our "mind." Kempf shows us that it takes place in our autonomic apparatus. The sacral division may be conditioned to need stimuli that are perverse or tabooed and cause irritability and depression until gratified, whereas their un-

[338]

restrained indulgence may greatly jeopardize the love for social esteem and the feeling of social fitness. The secret sense of social inferiority, due to some one's awareness of tabooed pelvic cravings, makes life in human society a fearful ordeal, which in turn, disturbs the respiratory, circulatory and gastronomic functions. Hence the needs or cravings of the different autonomic segments converge upon the projicient apparatus and behaviour is the physical or mechanical resultant. This compels the different autonomic segments to wage fierce conflict for control of our conduct and our conduct reveals the conflict.

That struggle grows fiercer as the civilization in which we live grows more complex. At birth, the autonomic apparatus works smoothly, because the infant is dependent upon the mother and hence irresponsible. But when the mother begins to train the infant to nurse, urinate and defecate under certain specific conditions, the autonomic apparatus for the first time clashes with society which insists on self-restraint, self-control and self-refinement.

Heedless indulgence by an individual of any age causes uncomfortable tensions in his associates, (disgust, fear, anger), and therefore they are compelled to control social tendencies in every individual from his earliest childhood.

[339]

Acquisitive cravings know no social law, however, and often threaten to jeopardize the personality by impelling it to do something which is illegal or immoral. For, after all, man is simply an ape that has learnt to wear clothes, to use words and signs and that can foresee in a general sense the possible biological and social results of certain indulgences.

Autonomic segments of the infant are then trained (conditioned) to react to certain stimuli, for instance, to certain vocal sounds and touches indicating the time for nursing, to signs and touches indicating disapproval of certain acts; the fear of losing certain agreeable stimuli gradually develops in him a certain degree of self-control.

Many cravings of an ungratifiable or unjustifiable nature, however, resist all attempts on the part of our environment to curb them. Compensatory strivings are then set in motion to prevent them, either from manifesting themselves or from being recognized in order that the organism may escape the concomitant fear. A state of fear induces malnutrition and impotence and hence would be destructive for the individual and the race.

When a craving is allowed to make the organism aware of its needs, but is not allowed to cause overt acts, it is said to be *suppressed*. When it is

[340]

not allowed to cause the organism to become aware of its needs, it may be said to have been *repressed*.

But neither suppression nor repression is synonymous with annihilation. Whether we remain in ignorance of the fact that a boiler is full of steam or simply disregard that fact, the steam is there, seeking an outlet and likely to create an abnormal one, unless a normal outlet is provided.

Repressed autonomic segments, like steam in a boiler, need but the slightest opportunity offered by the environment, or the slightest relaxation of the repressing forces to obtain control of the sensori-motor nervous system. We may suppress our disgust or anger to save appearances but we will at the same time, by remarks, by our very tone of voice or gestures, betray our real feelings; we will have dreams which picture the attempted or successful gratification of suppressed cravings.

The essential difference between most sane and insane people is that insane people cannot control their repressed cravings while sane people can. That is to say, when people become fatigued, toxic, dazed and can no longer control their repressed cravings, those cravings cause a form of behaviour which is termed insane.

As the human individual grows and develops, he gradually becomes able to control the activities of the various cravings with the exception, however, of the sexual cravings. When sexual cravings are normal, they are naturally justified and, under certain conditions, they are permitted socially to dominate our behaviour.

When the personality, on the other hand, considers sexual cravings as shameful inferiorities, either because they are perverse or because the personality has been educated in a prudish way, the individual becomes forced into a form of adjustment which is abnormal on account of the autonomic conflict it entails.

Whenever a violent conflict rages in our autonomic apparatus between acquisitive and avertive cravings, a neurosis ensues, or rather, the neurosis is the conflict. No constitutional predisposition is needed to bring about its onset. Life's experiences and the influence of our environment and associates are sufficient as determining factors.

Kempf does not accept Freud's theory as to the importance of sex (love) in the causation of neurotic disturbances. Any of the primary cravings, love, hate, hunger, shame, sorrow, fear or disgust may cause a neurosis under appropriate conditions.

The neurotic is suffering from cravings which he cannot allow to dominate his personality.

[342]

Those cravings are so often located in postural tensions of certain organs that they are probably consistent things even if they are not always discoverable.

A strong craving like the famishing influence of protracted hunger, which originates in the stomach, or the severe itching of an area of the skin, may finally determine all the adjustments of the entire personality and be felt over the entire body.

The result may be a severe struggle to eliminate the craving from the personality. Or the personality may resign itself to the domination of the craving and to a regression in which the individual enjoys tensions and images, fancies, delusions, hallucinations which simulate the craved reality.

On the basis of this conception of the personality, Kempf rejects entirely the usual classification of mental disturbances into neuroses, psycho-neuroses and psychoses. That classification is very unscientific and unbiological for it is based upon symptoms which may change under different conditions or under the care of different physicians. In many institutions, for example, the diagnosis "manic-depressive" tacitly means recoverable, while "dementia praecox" means incurable, so that if a dementia praecox patient shows a tendency to recovery he is reclassified as "manic-depressive."

Kempf's classification takes into account the nature of the patient's autonomic cravings and his attitude toward them. It is, therefore, essentially mechanistic and truly biological.

Every nervous disturbance is designated as a neurosis.

The neurosis is then, according to its duration, termed *acute, chronic* or *periodic.* The term *acute* is reserved for cases of less than a year's duration. *Chronic* is applied to cases having had more than a year's duration or which have had an insidious course for more than a year before the consultation. *Periodic* is applied to cases which have periodic or intermittent episodes or recurrences accompanying natural phenomena such as menstruation, pregnancy, marriage, death of a child, etc.

The neurosis is further qualified with regard to its mechanism, that is, the insight the patient has retained. The neurosis is *benign* when the patient recognizes that his distress or disease is due to the suppression of unjustifiable or ungratifiable cravings which are a part of his personality. The neurosis is *pernicious* when the patient refuses to attribute his trouble to a personal cause or wish, insists that it is due to an impersonal cause or a malicious influence and tends to hate any one who would attribute it to a personal source.

[344]

According to the mechanism of the autonomic conflict involved, neuroses are differentiated into five types:

The *suppression neuroses* are characterized by the fact that the patient is more or less conscious of the nature and effect upon himself of his ungratifiable cravings. For instance, a man may be affected by his love for a faithless, indifferent or dead woman; a soldier may be caught between two fears, that of death and that of a court martial, etc., and know that it causes him insomnia, headache, cardiac anxiety, diarrhoea, etc.

In *repression neuroses,* the individual tries to prevent the autonomic cravings from making themselves known and influencing his personality. A repressed fear may make a man blind or lame and he may feel convinced that an actual fall, bruise or wrench is responsible for his condition, because he has succeeded in making himself forget the cravings that are relieved by being blind or lame.

Compensation neuroses are characterized by a reflex effort to develop functions which will compensate for some organic or functional inferiority or keep an undesirable craving repressed, which is unconsciously causing fear. Very often the effort is adapted or designed to destroy or defeat en-

[345]

vironment factors which arouse the intolerable craving or oppose the compensation. Egotism, intolerance and exaggerated claims are typical of compensation neuroses.

Regression neuroses are just the opposite. The individual makes no effort to win or retain social esteem and regresses to a lower, childlike or infantile level, becoming apathetic, slovenly, irresponsible, often showing suicidal tendencies, and allowing the cravings to do as they please.

The regression may be a relatively benign episode of a few months' duration. It may in other cases be followed by a feeling of having died and passed through a rebirth, and also of having eliminated all the sinful cravings in order to begin life anew. This form of adjustment may work as long as the subject lives in a protected, non-competitive environment. Later, an eccentric overcompensation often takes place which eventually leads to another neurosis or a permanent deterioration of the personality.

In *dissociation neuroses*, the patient succeeds in keeping his undesirable cravings repressed until they finally become dissociated. The individual is then conscious of weird, distorted images, hallucinations of past sensations and experiences which seem to gratify the dissociated effect although they

[346]

horrify the individual. The individual is also dominated by unacceptable, mysterious obsessions, fears, compulsions and inspirations. There may be also severe visceral distress, motor disturbances, amnesia, etc.

The analytic treatment as mapped out by Kempf, consists in developing a transference, that is, giving the subject an apportunity to rely upon the altruistic judgment of some authoritative practitioner and enabling him to allow his repressions to make themselves conscious.

Kempf disagrees with Jung on the extent to which the transference should be used and he considers it essential in order to help the neurotic to become socially constructive. Only in that way can the analyst fulfil the mission in which the neurotic's parents failed.

After the subject succeeds in giving full expression to his repressed affects, those affects become assimilated with the personality and form an intimate part of it, instead of remaining uncontrollable, unconscious or mysterious factors. In that way the dissociated cravings which cause obsessions, phobias, mannerisms, compulsions, delusions, hallucinations, regressions, eccentric compensations and prejudices, are once more merged with the organism from which they had been ab-

[347]

normally separated and the functional distortion disappears.

The subject having acquired insight and being free from the fear of something within himself, becomes capable of making a sensible, practical adjustment.

When that readjustment is effected an intelligent use of the reconstructive, suggestive method seems to be most effective in giving the neurotic new interests for which to live and work, without seeking abnormal compensations for prudish or fearful repressions or yielding to perverse cravings.

The choice of a method, Kempf thinks, should be left to the patient but he should not be allowed to avoid the work of reconstruction. Furthermore, the analysis should be accompanied by vigorous indulgence in social play requiring exposure of functional or organic inferiorities to more or less critical evaluation by competitors. Thus the subject will become immune to the fear of failure or inferiority and will avoid eccentric compensation and a seclusive mode of life.

BIBLIOGRAPHY

To understand Kempf's works one must have acquired a good working knowledge of the autonomic system and of endocrinology. See the bibliography following the

[348]

chapter on Nerves and Nervousness. Kempf's style is extremely technical and remarkable for its accuracy but not easily understood by the layman. The body of his doctrines is contained in his book "Psychopathology," published by C. V. Mosby, in which he discusses the physical basis of the personality, the psychology of the family, the universal struggle for virility, organic and functional inferiorities and their influence on the personality, the various forms of neuroses, etc.

Also consult the following monographs and articles:

KEMPF, EDWARD J.—"The Mechanistic Classification of Neuroses and Psychoses Produced by Distortion of the Autonomic-affective Functions," *Journal of Nervous and Mental Disease*, August, 1919.

KEMPF, EDWARD J.—"The Tonus of Autonomic Segments as Causes of Abnormal Behaviour,"*Journal of Nervous and Mental Disease*, January, 1920.

KEMPF, EDWARD J.—"The Autonomic Functions and the Personality," *Nervous and Mental Disease Monograph Series* No. 28.

INDEX

Index

[352]

[353]